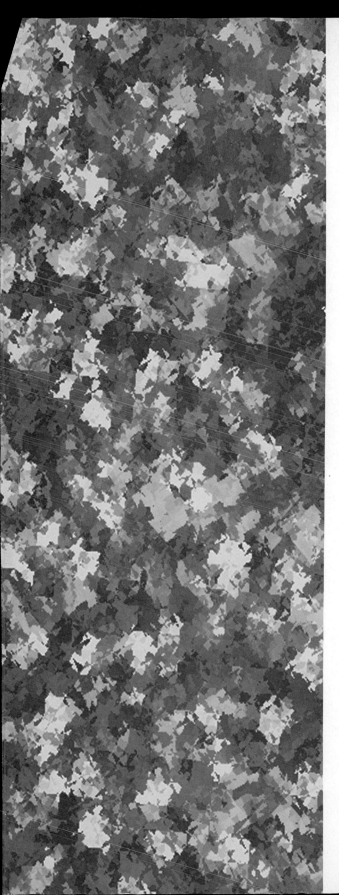

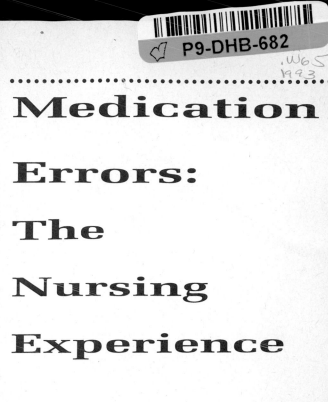
Medication Errors: The Nursing Experience

Zane Robinson Wolf Phd, RN, FAAN

Professor of Nursing, School of Nursing,
LaSalle University and Associate
Director of Nursing for Research,
Albert Einstein Medical Center

D Delmar Publishers Inc.™

I T P™

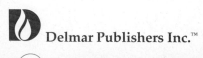

Notice to the Reader

Publisher does not warrant or guarantee any of the products described herein or perform any independent analysis in connection with any of the product information contained herein. Publisher does not assume, and expressly disclaims, any obligation to obtain and include information other than that provided to it by the manufacturer.

The reader is expressly warned to consider and adopt all safety precautions that might be indicated by the activities described herein and to avoid all potential hazards. By following the instructions contained herein, the reader willingly assumes all risks in connection with such instructions.

The publisher makes no representations or warranties of any kind, including but not limited to, the warranties of fitness for particular purpose or merchantability, nor are any such representations implied with respect to the material set forth herein, and the publisher takes no responsibility with respect to such material. The publisher shall not be liable for any special, consequential or exemplary damages resulting, in whole or in part, from the readers' use of, or reliance upon, this material.

Cover Credit: J^2 Designs

Delmar staff:
Publisher: David C. Gordon
Senior Acquisitions Editor: Bill Burgower
Assistant Editor: Debra M. Flis
Project Editor: Danya M. Plotsky
Production Coordinator: Barbara A. Bullock
Art and Design Coordinators: Timothy J. Conners
                              Megan K. DeSantis

For information, address

Delmar Publishers Inc.
3 Columbia Circle, Box 15015
Albany, NY 12212–5015

Printed in the United States of America
Published simultaneously in Canada by Nelson Canada,
a division of The Thomson Corporation

  2 3 4 5 6 7 8 9 10 XXX 00 99 98 97 96 95 94

Library of Congress Cataloging-in-Publication Data

Wolf, Zane Robinson.
   Medication errors: the nursing experience / Zane Robinson Wolf.
      p.   cm. — (RealNursing series)
   Includes bibliographical references.
   ISBN 0–8273–6262–5
   1. Medication errors. 2. Nursing. I. Title.
II. Series.
   [DNLM: 1. Medication Errors — nurses' instruction. 2. Drug Therapy
   — adverse effects — nurses' instruction. QZ 42 W855m]
RM146.W65 1993
615.5'8 — dc20
DNLM/DLC   93-5886
for Library of Congress   CIP

REALNURSING SERIES
Alice M. Stein, MA, RN, Series Editor
Medical College of Pennsylvania

HEALING YOURSELF: A NURSE'S GUIDE TO SELF-CARE AND RENEWAL

COMMUNICATION AND IMAGE IN NURSING

FEAR AND AIDS/HIV: EMPATHY AND COMMUNICATION

SEXUAL HEALTH: A NURSE'S GUIDE

20 LEGAL PITFALLS FOR NURSES TO AVOID

TO LISTEN, TO COMFORT, TO CARE: REFLECTIONS ON DEATH AND DYING

THE NURSE AS HEALER

MEDICATION ERRORS: THE NURSING EXPERIENCE

FUTURE TITLES:

CRITICAL BUSINESS SKILLS FOR NURSES

HEALING ALCOHOL AND SUBSTANCE ABUSE

ETHICAL DILEMMAS IN NURSING

WAR STORIES: DIFFICULT NURSING DECISIONS

THE FEMINIST NURSE

THE GAY AND LESBIAN NURSE

INTERVENTIONS IN EVERYDAY NURSING EMERGENCIES

HEALING RACISM IN NURSING

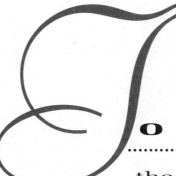o

the nurses from the North, South, East, and West who shared their stories

$\mathcal{J}$able of Contents

....

PART III
MEDICATION ERRORS AND CHEMICALLY
DEPENDENT NURSES

PART IV
SEEKING SOLUTIONS

10. A Model of Nurse-Made Medication Errors ∎ 137

11. Nurses' Mistakes at Work: An Essay ∎ 141

PART V
APPENDIXES

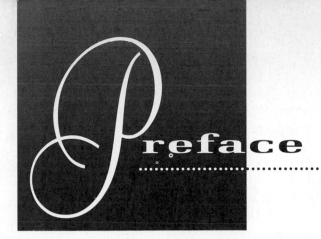

Preface

Hospital nurses are committed to giving their patients the safest care possible, especially in relation to medication administration. So when they make medication errors, as every nurse almost inevitably does, they confront one of their worst fears: harming patients. This book is written for all nurses who administer medications to patients, who fear making medication errors, and who make medication errors.

In this book, nurses share their experiences and provide useful suggestions on dealing with medication errors. Ideally, this advice will help other nurses in their efforts to reduce the incidence of medication errors and to restrict the degree of harm resulting from such errors. In addition, suggestions are provided to help nurses reduce the incidence of medication errors through a test of risks and dosage calculation skills and an instructional booklet aimed at reducing the risks associated with medication errors and preventing errors from occurring.

This book also presents recommendations to clinicians and managers interested in decreasing medication errors. The content in the book is based on qualitative research studies conducted by the author. Phenomenological interviewing, semistructured interviewing, and focus-group approaches were used to elicit nurses' stories on their experiences with medication errors.

Administrators of departments of nursing, nurse managers, assistant nurse managers, staff nurses, risk managers, quality assurance directors, physicians, pharmacists, hospital lawyers, hospital administrators, patients, and patients' family members and friends regard medication errors seriously. Even if clinical symptoms do not provide evidence of any harm caused by such mistakes, the occurrence of an error nevertheless serves as a warning and places health care workers on alert. Hospital workers only reluctantly admit making medication errors. Because hospital personnel fear litigation, nurses seldom disclose the stories of their errors and those of their nurse colleagues. This book contains those stories—the accounts of nurses' experiences when they made medication errors. They provide an inside view of nurses' work and explore the impact of medication-related mistakes on nurses in the context of the American hospital. I hope that nurses will gain a deeper understanding of and an expanded perspective regarding the repercussions of medication errors on many departments in hospitals and on many levels of nurses within nursing service organizations. By reading this book, both nursing students and practicing nurses will be helped to become more sensitive to the complex issues associated with medication errors. They may benefit from self-administering the test on risks associated with medication errors and studying Appendix C.

Chapters 1 through 4 (Part I) are primarily personal accounts of nurse-made medication errors and an analysis of sixteen nurses' experiences with making these errors. Chapters 5 and 6 (Part II) contain practical approaches and advice regarding medication errors that are provided by staff nurses, nurse managers, nurse administrators, quality assurance coordinators, and a risk manager. In Part III, another perspective is explored. Nurse managers' and nurse administrators' accounts of their experiences with chemically dependent nurses are examined in Chapter 7. In Chapter 8, a nurse administrator provides an account of narcotics' being diverted from patient units. Part IV focuses on the search for solutions to the problem of medication errors. General advice on reducing risks associated with medication errors is given in Chapter 9, and a model of medication errors is described in Chapter 10.

The appendixes include a reference list and two research proposals focused on the problem of medication errors. The first study includes a test of risks related to medication errors and drug calculation problems. A teaching plan and instructional booklet are also included. The second study, a descriptive one, attempts to predict harm to patients following medication errors, using data generated from nurses' responses to an instrument called the Medication Error Risk Profile.

The nurses who shared their stories came from different regions of the United States. I am deeply indebted to them. I thank also the following supporters of my efforts: Charles, Jessica, Zana, and Kerrin Wolf; Rita Jablonski, Elaine Volk, and Terry McGoldrick who worked with me on the studies in Appendix A; and Mary Segal and John Whyte for their helpful critique of the first study. This book represents my interpretations of nurses' stories and should not be attributed to anyone else.

Introduction

Nurses who work in hospitals consistently act to maintain patient safety, but sometime in their career they may make a mistake at work that may jeopardize the safety of a patient. Medication errors are unintentional mistakes associated with drugs and intravenous (IV) solutions that are made during the prescription, transcription, dispensing, and administration phases of drug preparation and distribution. They occur when nurses administer drugs to patients, notwithstanding the procedures, routines, policies, and rituals designed to eliminate errors through specific safeguards.

Hospital-based nurses work persistently and earnestly to eliminate drug errors. Nurse educators also support a long-time commitment to protect patients from medication errors as they initiate nursing students into the art and skill of medication administration. Many nurses assume their share of the responsibility—along with physicians, pharmacists, risk managers, hospital administrators, medical clerks, and patients—to reduce and eliminate these mistakes. Drug errors implicate health care personnel associated with these mistakes at hospitals. They participate in the complex series of events that comprise the activities of medication administration and that accompany errors. It is difficult, and perhaps impossible, to eradicate random medication errors by prospective actions. However, the causes of systematic errors can be identified and addressed prospectively in an effort to reduce the rate of medication errors on patient units.

Nurses usually accept the seriousness of their responsibility in relation to medication errors. Many of these errors are publicly aired through the avenues of change-of-shift reports, incident reports, gossip, and nursing staff meetings; others go unreported; some are discussed only in confidence with nurse colleagues, who may acknowledge fears of also making medication errors. Nurses highly value proficiency and safety in giving medications. When they make medication errors, they may feel as if they have failed. Some nurses are embarrassed by these mistakes and avoid discussing an error when it is made. If the patient who is not administered medication correctly appears to suffer no harm, the error may go unreported. Time may reduce but never eliminate the guilt associated with the medication errors nurses report and consider to be serious. Many years later, most nurses are able to recollect vividly and describe certain medication errors.

Acknowledging these experiences can assist nurses in understanding their meaning. Specific accounts of medication errors made by nurses are not often published. The nurses who decided to share their stories in this book hope that others may learn from them. Also, understanding medication errors from the perspective of nurses' experiences may help to explain the private actions nurses may perform when they discover that they have made a mistake. These may include surreptitiously checking the patient's vital signs; calling the patient's unit from home to check on the patient's status; or frequently checking how the patient looks (color of skin, depth of respiration, and so on).

The phenomenon of mistakes made at work is not unique to nurses. According to sociologist E. C. Hughes, people working in all occupations make these errors and suffer a great deal of anxiety as a result. Often they do not discuss the risks associated with work-related mistakes and exert themselves to keep their skills well developed in order to eliminate errors. Medication errors constitute a special type of mistake. Medications or IVs containing medications are either not administered or are administered in a manner other than prescribed. The workers who make these errors are frequently professionals working in health-care institutions who implicitly uphold the ethical principle of doing no harm to their patients. Because of this commitment, nurses and other caregivers typically react with feelings of horror when they make medication errors.

In the past, nurses may have believed that if they did not document medication errors, no one would take action against them. But in a case in the early 1980s, the court ruled "that the statute of limitations begins at the time of the discovery of the injury or death. . . . Thus an incident can be investigated long after it occurs" (Gardner, 1987, p. 188). In spite of a personal reluctance to report medication errors, most nurses and others involved with these mistakes recognize the need for vigilance and for truthfulness about what happened at the time an error was discovered and what was done to prevent patient injury. Not only is unnecessary harm avoided because of effective interventions following the error, but malpractice litigation begins with a better defense. Acknowledging responsibility for the error is considered the best action to take. Nevertheless, some nurses still do not report their errors.

In many ways, nurses have shouldered their responsibility concerning medication errors. They have instituted monitoring programs to document errors and the reasons for their occurrence. They have worked with other hospital personnel to develop methods designed to reduce systems errors resulting from flaws in the construction and implementation of hospital procedures or in the design of medication prescription, administration, and dispensing systems. Yet no one has identified a system that will eliminate all drug errors (although primary nursing using unit-dose dispensing has allowed nurses to monitor drug errors better).

Quality assurance (QA) programs monitor medication errors in hospitals and other health care institutions. The results of QA studies serve to alert staff nurses and their administrative colleagues to problems on patient units. For example, error rates are used as indicators of quality patient care and are considered worthy of close scrutiny. Some authors hold that decreased rates of medication errors influence patient length of stay and hospital costs (Jonville et al, 1991). There are reports that the use of an improved medication error report form improves data collection. Based on these data, different solutions are instituted to reduce error rates. Some nurses caution that nursing staff must be carefully approached by nursing supervisors and administrators if error rates increase because of better documentation. Nurses may fail to report errors as a response to rising rates.

Other health care professionals may blame these errors on nurses' lack of efficiency. They may charge that deficits in motivation, training, and individual nurse ability adversely influence performance and result in drug errors.

Two studies associate stress with increased errors. In a prospective study of accident and error rates, recent life changes and stresses, social support, state of depression, illness rate, and coping skills were measured in nursing students at the beginning and end of a five-week period. The most powerful predictors of students' accident and error rates were the number of life changes two years before the error and the amount of social support available to help students cope. Equally important is the explanation given in a study comparing the effect on medication error rates of primary medication administration (where primary and associate nurses give medications to their patients in a district) versus functional medication administration (where the nurse gives medications to the entire unit). The increased stress level among nurses, resulting from a heavier than usual load of acutely ill patients, may have influenced a higher rate of medication errors.

That many errors are not detected or are not reported might imply that nurses fear the personal consequences of these mistakes. Nurses generally are unwilling to report omission or wrong-time errors unless a potent medication was involved. For some, medication errors may be equivalent to failure. The possibility of harming patients in spite of the best therapeutic intentions can cause personal discomfort. Drug errors can be very stressful for nurses for many reasons; however, there are few studies exploring the experience and its meaning for nurses. One nurse has provided a beginning exploration on how neonatal intensive care unit (NICU) nurses create meaning in their stressful work with critically ill babies, including when they make medication errors. According to Sally Hutchinson, nurses reconstruct the reality of the NICU through personal and shared meanings and are able to accept the value of their difficult work. They are horrified if they make a medication error when caring for a critically ill baby.

When nurses acknowledge making medication errors and other clinical mistakes, their disclosure and remorse are interpreted to mean that they care for the patient. Otherwise they would not have accepted responsibility for the mistake and sacrificed personal self-comfort. However, colleagues consider a nurse's repeated pattern of mistakes to be very serious. The delinquent nurse may be asked to resign.

Nurses who recognize and accept their role in medication errors usually correct themselves and move on to other potentially hazardous clinical work where mistakes are a possibility. But medication errors remain in every nurse's memory.

REFERENCES

Gardner, C. (1987). Risk management of medication errors. *NITA*, May–June, pp. 187–196.

Hughes, E. C. (1951). Mistakes at work. *Journal of Economics and Political Science, 17*, pp. 320–327.

Jonville, A. E., Autret, E., Bavvux, F., Berkrand, P. P., Barbier, P., and Gauchez, A. M. (1991). Characteristics of medication errors in pediatrics. *DICP, The Annals of Pharmacotherapy, 25*, pp. 1113–1117.

Part I

Nurses' Experiences Making Medication Errors

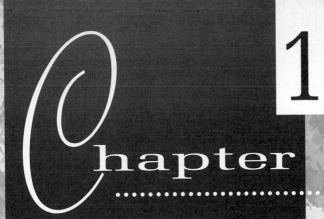

Chapter 1

Making a Medication Error as a Nursing Student

Nursing students quickly learn the personal and professional dangers of making medication errors. Their fears of these mistakes are augmented by the stories other nurses share about what happened to them or their friends while still enrolled in nursing school.

An experienced registered nurse shared her account of making a medication error when she was a senior in college. Her first thought was that she was going to be expelled from the nursing program.

I PULLED OUT THE WRONG ONE!

I was a senior in college. It was the second semester, and we probably had six or eight weeks left to graduation, and this was our leadership group. We had our clinical experience at a large hospital and were on wards of about 60 patients. I was giving all the medications to all those patients.

The patients had to line up outside the medication room for their pain medicine, and the nurses had to do all the preoperative medications, plus the routine ones. I was called for a pre-op medication. It was written as Nembutal, and, of course, the drugs were labeled pentyl and phenobarbital, and I pulled out the wrong one—phenobarbital instead of pentyl. I didn't realize it until I came back to the nurses' station after I had given the medication and sent the patient down to the OR [operating room]. I came out to sign out the drugs and all of a sudden felt this white-hot dagger. It was like, "Oh, my God! I pulled out the wrong one!"

The thing that bothered me the most was my initial instinct: I did not want to tell anyone because I couldn't imagine what was going to happen. It probably didn't take that long, but it seemed like forever before I decided that I had to tell somebody. It was probably just by the time I signed my name to the wrong stuff and realized that I had to do this. Well, the head nurse was a man, and he was pretty brusque with me—understandably so, I guess. I knew that I had made a life-threatening mistake—that this was really a horrible thing. The head nurse sent me downstairs to talk to the anesthesiologist before I spoke to my instructor.

My face matched my white uniform; there was no color in my lips; I was a mess. The anesthesiologist said, "I can tell just from looking at you that you'll never, ever make that mistake again." Once he knew that I had given the short-acting instead of the long-acting drug, he could compensate for it—and he was pleased that I came down in time so that he could compensate.

Then I had the horrible job of going to tell my instructor before I told anyone else. I thought that this was a big enough mistake that I would be expelled from school just eight weeks from graduation. What would I do? How could I tell my parents? How would I live this down? No one would accept me now in their program because of this stupid mistake. I was really concerned about what was going to happen to me.

As it turned out, the nursing instructors talked about the error in class so every student would know that this kind of mistake happens, and they gave advice about what to do about it. I wished that the floor would open and swallow me up. I was positive that I was the only one who had even done that before. But I was also thinking that the humiliation was a lot better than being expelled from school. I'll take the humiliation, I decided. I thought about how our class had started with 75 students, and we graduated 52.

I remained pretty nervous about my mistake, and so I was relieved and happy when I graduated and then passed the state board examination. At that point I decided that I was not so bad after all—but I was still pretty nervous about the drug error.

The medication error made me really feel inadequate—that I wasn't a good nurse, that good nurses don't make mistakes, that I shouldn't have been pressured by all these people outside the door waiting for their pain medicine, that I was foolish, that I acted too quickly, that I really should have taken more time in checking before I went on to the next medication.

To this day, it is still embarrassing to think that I made such a big mistake. It was especially upsetting since I was in school and supposed to be so careful about everything. And as a senior nursing student, I was on my own by that time.

I still can't believe that I made that mistake. Now whenever I give medications, I check the bottle twice before I do anything.

Looking back, I think that I was probably cocky before making the error. After I realized what I had done, I was mortified and couldn't believe that I had done such a horrible thing. How was I going to face up to it, and how could I cover it up?

I couldn't cover it up; it was too harmful a thing to cover up. Later, it still was an embarrassing situation to remember. I had done a stupid thing, and I had to be careful because it's easy to make stupid mistakes. When you make stupid mistakes, peoples' lives are at stake. I think that this single incident made me more careful with medications.

I talked to the nursing supervisor and the head nurse about what I had done, but I think that the anesthesiologist was the biggest comfort. He really helped me resolve the fact that this error was correctable. If I hadn't told him, things might not have been as easy for the patient in the OR.

My nursing instructor was at first accepting of the error, but I was pretty mortified when she discussed it in class. I didn't know that she was going to do that. We had already talked about the error in our post conference, but it was a smaller group and so that was easier. But in front of all 50 classmates, it was pretty rough.

The medication error is clear in my mind even though it happened 15 years ago. I can still see the whole room. I can see the patients standing outside and waiting for their pain medications. I even know what uniform I was wearing—the cap and everything. The patient was on one of the 20-bed wards on that unit, which also had some private rooms. The hospital is pretty well emblazoned in my brain too. I remember every inch of that place. I remember looking into the metal narcotic box and seeing the medication cart that we used to pass out medications. I knew that I probably wasn't sure enough just to yank something out of the box. I should have looked the medication up, but I didn't take the time. That's what really stands out in my mind: I should have taken the time to look it up.

After that medication error, I was much more cautious and a lot slower. It's not as rote as it was before. You may get cocky about what you do before you make a mistake, and then you do something horrible, and you're really careful for a long time.

You're really supposed to be doing everything right as a student; you're not supposed to make mistakes until you're out on your own. I guess it made me really believe that I was an honest person after all. What upset me the most was my initial response: "Oh, my God! I can't tell anybody that I did this!" That was what scared me the most and made me think that I wasn't an honest person. But actually coming through and saying, "Oh, God, I really made this mistake—you have to help me out of this," made me realize my honesty.

My initial reaction was to cover up the medication error. I don't know whether other people have ever had that reaction. I told everybody that I had tried to cover it up because that was the most embarrassing part of it. I don't think this reaction lasted long, but it was long enough to scare me.

I don't think I've ever really gotten over it. The mistake is still fresh in my memory.

Summary

Nursing instructors must consider each nursing student's right to confidentiality when medication errors are made. The public exposure in the classroom may humiliate an already upset student. Rather than the approach described here, it is better if nursing professors acknowledge the inevitability of mistakes in all human endeavors. They should encourage students to report errors and to document them carefully. Above all else, patient safety must be the nursing student's and the professional nurse's focus.

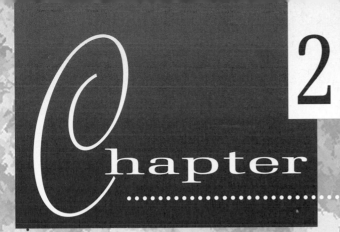

Chapter 2

Making a Medication Error as a Graduate Nurse

In this chapter, four recently graduated nurses recall their medication errors. The first two made the errors within a few months of the interview; the third nurse had made the errors years before describing it.

A PREDICTION BECOMES REALITY

That medication error is the easiest thing in the world to describe! And I'll tell you one thing, it feels better talking about it, especially knowing that it happens to everybody else.

The night that it happened, I didn't realize what I had done until about an hour and a half later. And when I did realize, it was kind of like that fight-or-flight syndrome. The adrenaline flowed, only it was more like nerves; I was really nervous and really hot. And I said, "Did I really do that? Did I really do that?" When I realized that I made the error, I called my preceptor since I was still on orientation. She was very calming and relaxing and told me, "It happens to everybody. It will be all right. We'll take care of it. We'll call up the physician. We'll write an incident report. Everything will be all right." But I still felt like an idiot. How could I do that? I don't care how many people it happens to, it shouldn't have happened to me. That's how I felt.

I worried about the patient all night. I looked in on him every 5 minutes. It was insulin I had administered incorrectly, and I took his blood sugar every hour. Anyway, everything turned out to be OK. Then about a week later, the attending physician came up. I didn't have that patient, but he happened to come in and he said, "Did anybody have this patient?" I replied, "No, but what's the problem?" "Oh," he said, "I just wanted to know what happened the other night with the insulin." I felt my face get so red because nobody really had to know about it—although I wanted to tell everybody. I think the more people I tell, the better I feel. If I kept it inside, I would not be comfortable. Another nurse told me that sometimes that can happen: you can keep a medication error inside. But I can't imagine doing that because of the guilt that I felt. I was scared to death. When I realized that it happens and everything is OK, I was fine, but when this attending physician asked, "What happened the other night?" I relived the mistake. My face got red, and I started steaming up. I said, "Let's talk about this outside."

I'll tell you one thing: I'll never make that mistake again. After making that error, I triple-check syringes and make sure that I have the exact amount. I look at it and go back and check the orders. I triple-check everything now; get all my pills out—get everything out that I need, then look at it, check the order, look at it, check the order. That's how I do it now. I am much, much more aware of what I'm doing.

Right before making the error, I was trying to get organized because it was my first night on evenings. As a graduate nurse, I was terribly unorganized; I have improved since then. I was in and out of every room, and it just happened.

The fact that I made an error didn't hit me until after I had given the medication. If it had hit me right before I gave it, I would have thanked my lucky stars. But when I realized what I had done, the first thing that ran through my mind was that I had to tell somebody immediately. It couldn't wait. I just had the feeling that my stomach dropped. I was worried to death about the patient all night.

The first thing I did was take the patient's blood sugar. It was 64—or something like that—so I gave him crackers and juice. Then I called my preceptor, and she told me that I had to call the physician who was covering him. My preceptor worked the same schedule that I did, and she came right over to help me.

I talked to someone else about the error. I had to tell the person whom I was giving a report to, so I took her aside and told her what had happened. She said to me, "Well, I did the same thing. And, you know, it happens to everybody." She knew that I had made a medication error as I was telling her and finished what I was saying. Just knowing that it had happened to her too and that it wasn't such a—I mean, it *is* a big deal. God forbid it should have been potassium or something. I could have killed him, and that's why I still think about it sometimes now.

I went home that night, and I don't think I slept a wink. I don't think I slept for nights after that. The next day I didn't want to go to work because everyone was going to know about it. I asked myself why it had to happen. The next night I worked was a Wednesday night, and I was organized. I checked and double-checked and triple-checked my orders.

I just had to keep telling myself that everything was OK. Thank God that the patient had a high blood sugar at the time this happened. And thank God that it was insulin and not something else, because with insulin, I gave him crackers, and the blood sugar came right back up to a nice level, so everything was OK. I thank God that everything was OK because I had somebody's life in my hands.

When I was at the beginning of my orientation, everyone told us that we would have a medication error—that it happens to everybody—and they told us what we had to do. At the time, I thought that this was not going to happen to me. I checked three times; I triple-checked. That was what they taught us at school—that you have to keep checking it and checking it. But in spite of my checking, it happened!

My preceptor made the whole medication error experience easy for me. She said to me, "Well, it's good that you're telling everybody about it. You know, there are some people who would let an error go unreported." I could have decided not to report the error. I could have loaded the patient up with sugar, but I would not have been able to live with myself. I'm a very honest person. I would have had a terrible time. The guilt was phenomenal. I have a hard time dealing with guilt, and that night, after I got it off my chest and started telling everybody, I just had to deal with what I had done.

That night, I was terrified. I'm the type of person where nothing is a major big deal, but that night I felt as if it was. I felt that I had to take care of this error. I sweated and was so nervous. But after I talked to my preceptor, I felt better. She was so calm and relaxed and put her arm around me. She assured me, "Oh, it's going to be all right." We sat down and completed the incident report together. She said, "You don't have to tell anybody about it." I told the night shift about it, and the more people I told, the better I felt. The more people who knew about it and the more people who said, "Oh yeah, that happened to me too, that's nothing," the better I felt.

My name is not even on the incident report. My preceptor filled it out and signed her name to it. I put a little note in the chart—how much insulin given and so on, and I wrote down all his blood sugars that I took.

It just takes time to work it out with yourself, even though everything was all right. I really felt better when the patient was discharged. Seeing him every day and having him as a patient every day was difficult. *He* thought that I was the most wonderful nurse on the floor. He didn't know what had happened. He just knew, "Well, my blood sugar is running a little low. That's why they're taking my sugar all of the time."

The most difficult part was filling out the incident report, because I had to relive the error, and at that time, I didn't want to think about it. I wanted to take the patient's blood sugar every 5 minutes. I wanted to be with my patient. I didn't want to keep reliving it again and again by completing the incident report.

Everyone was really understanding, even the resident physician who was covering the patient. I thought that others would think, "What an idiot this person is. Look at what she did." But nobody was like that to me, and nobody treated me as if I was an idiot. It was just something that happened.

I was scared to death. I will never, ever give insulin wrong again without thinking of that error. I couldn't sleep that night. The medication error was really hard to deal with. It took some time. I'm fine with it now. But I think about it every time I take somebody's blood sugar or give insulin. I look at it and look at it, and look at it.

PROCEEDING WITH CAUTION

It was a right medication—right dose—wrong route error. I was in a hurry. I had to get done on time for my ride at 11:30. I didn't have a car because I had been in a little accident three or four weeks before, and my sister-in-law was going to pick me up. She had to drop me off at my house, and that meant that she had to come back to the city, because she lives there. And I had a lot on my mind: what kind of a car I was going to get, and why the insurance company wasn't settling the accident—I needed the money to buy a new car.

I realized that I made an error immediately after I signed out the medication. I put "PO," which is by mouth, and then my initial. Then I went back again and I saw it: IV. That's when I realized that it was an error. I gave the medication by the wrong route.

I felt a great deal of fear about the situation, for my job and my career. I thought about how I had worked hard—four years in school—and now it was down the drain. I worried about what I was going to do. I stood for about 10 seconds, trying to think of people I had to contact or things that I had to do. I wondered whether I could do anything about it but, of course, I couldn't, so I decided that I had to try to compose myself and my thinking. I had to go to the right people.

After I realized what had happened and thought about what I should do and what I could do to erase that error completely—not erase it literally but do something that would not indicate in black and white that I made an error—I ran to one of the other nurses, and she told me to cross it out and write IV instead of PO.

I tried to argue with her that I didn't think that was right. I had made an error and could not cover myself and my mistake by doing what she said—crossing PO out and writing IV in. I told her that I was not going to learn anything by doing what she told me to do. I'd be cheating myself and was not going to cheat. I made an error, and I wanted to get some feedback about it. I didn't want to be punished for that mistake and refused to think that I would get punished, but if that was the last resort, I was going to accept that.

Honestly, my feeling at that time was that I was ready to be fired. That's what my coordinator saw in me too. I was shaking and was really scared, for two reasons: What was going to happen to the patient and what was going to happen to my job. Those were the two main things. I didn't even know about the embarrassment that would follow for my family and my friends.

The first person I discussed the error with was the other staff nurse. I had paged the supervisor, but there was no answer, so I tried the first person I saw, in case she knew something—maybe an antidote for that medication or something that I didn't know. I discussed the whole thing with her. I told her that I did not realize that I had made an error until I saw the order for the IV on the cardex.

When I discussed the error with the supervisor, I felt different. I was petrified about what I had to tell her, but after I started telling her, I read her eyes and told her everything. I felt better even though I did not know what was going to happen.

The doctor was the least concerned. I said I made an error; he had ordered an IV medication, and I gave it PO. He said, "Oh, you wanted to change it to PO?" And I asked myself, "And you were worried!" I laughed after that. And then they were all laughing at me—the supervisor too. I said, "What an idiot." That's what I said.

After I talked to these people and to my clinical coordinator, I felt better. But still, it's in my mind. I cannot get rid of that—the error that I made. What if something happened to the patient? It's my responsibility; it's my error. My clinical coordinator told me that I was being too hard on myself.

A few days after I made the error, I was trying to remember the incident. I cursed myself and said, "You've seen it. It's right there." Except for that time, I always double-check the orders and the cardex and the medication. For about three weeks after that, I kept asking myself why

I had made that error and how I had made it. I didn't get an answer.

I'm much more careful about giving medications, and I think I've gained a lot of confidence in myself to do more. I feel it's more challenging now because of the error. They're expecting more errors; the supervisors told me that. I want to prove to them that I will not make a second error. I cannot just take safety for granted. If I'm working, I have to concentrate on my work—not think about anything but what I'm doing at that particular moment. I promised myself that if there's going to be any interruption, even for 5 seconds, or for 10 seconds, or 1 or 2 minutes, I'm going to get out and go someplace else—the break room, the bathroom, or someplace like that—to get rid of the distraction. I'll take my time. I don't care if I have to stay for 3 extra hours without getting paid. I don't care.

Talking to the supervisors, other nurses, and especially the doctor made the medication error easier. Now I know that medications are my weakness, and that is where I am concentrating.

The doctor's comment made me feel better. When I got home, I reflected, "The doctor doesn't care. Why should I?" But after I said that, I said, "I should care." And I did.

The lesson that I learned from this error is that it is very easy to make errors when giving medications with all these heavy assignments and patients with high acuity levels. I'm new, and I'm still learning, and I know I'm going to be making mistakes. I always keep that in mind in order to remind myself that I am subject to errors. I have to be careful. That is the only thing to remember.

I'm still a little worried about my nursing career because my superior knows about the error. I don't know if it's in my record. They told me that it's not, but I'm not sure. I have goals for my career. I'm planning to pursue a doctorate, or at least a master's degree, and that's the thing I'm worrying about. Will the medication error affect my reputation as a nurse, considering that I just started working here?

I guess they had a meeting about the error, because they were really concerned about it. They said that I did a good thing when I reported my mistake. I felt very proud of this whole floor. When the incoming shift came in, I could have hidden it from them. They noticed right away that I was worried and that something was wrong, so I told the person I gave the report to about the error. She was really worried about me, so she talked to the clinical coordinator and asked her to talk to me.

The following day, the clinical coordinator called me, and I was scared; I thought, "This is it! The pink slip is here." We sat down, and I asked, "What did you want to talk to me about?" Her answer was, "Well, chill out." Then I said, "And . . . ?" I was waiting for the termination letter that she would hand me. She was holding a letter, and I thought that was it. Instead she said, "Look, you're a great nurse. You did the right thing; you went to the right people; you recognized your mistake. That's what makes a great nurse." And I felt great about it—not that it stopped me from taking the opportunity to think about the error I made. I'm still thinking about it. I think it will stay in my mind for as long as I am a nurse.

A CASCADE OF MEDICATION ERROR MEMORIES

The first medication error I remember was when I was a new graduate. I was working in the old building in this hospital, and I had given histamine to a patient who had some sort of vasculitis. They wanted to give her histamine to stimulate some sort of a response—for migraines, I think it was. The pharmacy sent up five vials of histamine phosphate base, and I had given all five vials, for a total of 1 milligram of histamine. It actually turned out not to be an error, but at the time I thought it was. I thought I had given five times the dosage. Well, I was afraid. I thought this woman could have an anaphylactic reaction and die. I could have killed her.

I was beside myself. I was absolutely mortified, first of all, because I had made a mistake. I was terrified for the patient, thinking that I could have killed her—that she was going to have this horrible reaction. It was the worst day of my life.

Another medication error happened when I was in nursing school and I hung the wrong bottle of hyperal [hyperalimentation]. I thought it was the worst tragedy of my lifetime. I thought, "Oh, my God," because I worked at another hospital then. I had worked with those nurses when I was a nurse's aide, and I was thinking, "Oh, my God, they're going to think I'm terrible." And then, of course, there was all the fear associated with hanging the wrong hyperalimentation bottle. It was the right patient but the wrong bottle number. I remember being so totally mortified. All things considered, it turned out all right. One IV had trace elements in it, and the other one didn't have vitamins.

I guess when I put it in perspective, it wasn't that bad, but at the time, I thought it was the worst thing in the world. The other nurses weren't really upset, but I remember the horrible feeling. I was thinking, "Oh, my God, I'm terrible!" It was terrible because I had made a mistake, and it could have hurt the patient. The feeling that you could have hurt somebody was awful. It turned out that I didn't—and that's the way it is with a lot of medication errors. But the fact remained that something like that could have been a problem.

After I saw that I had made the error, I knew horror. That's probably the best word.

Immediately afterward, I tried to figure out where I had gone wrong. What had I done? What could I do now that I made the mistake? What should I do so that it would never happen again? I thought about double-checking dosages, making sure the orders were written clearly, and that kind of thing. I knew that I must double-check everything and take my time with everything. I tried not to rush giving medications. If it was a medication that I wasn't sure about, I called the pharmacy or someone else before I gave it and said, "What is this?"

The easiest part of the experience was the reassurance that it wasn't such a horrible mistake. The lady didn't die. Just knowing that the patient didn't suffer was probably the best thing. The most difficult part of making the error was the fact that I made a mistake, and it was a stupid one.

What made me report the error was the possible severity of it. If you hang the wrong IV—if you give potassium or something like that—you report it. Sometimes if you are late, you have a tendency not to report the error. If there are peak and trough levels that get missed, you technically should report the error. If you don't always chart an IV site or a medication site, you tend not to write things up that you should.

I was involved in another medication error recently that was chemo [chemotherapy]. This woman was a teacher, and she wanted her treatments Friday afternoon, late. That was her control piece; she wanted it at that time, and she wouldn't get to the hospital until 4:30 or 5:00. We all wanted to leave because it was Friday afternoon. She would come every week. She was supposed to get 5-FU (fluorouracil; antimetabolite) and methotrexate (antimetabolite).

The day of the error, I was giving her the injection, and her hands started to burn. I had never known that to occur before, but the syringe was labeled 500 milligrams of 5-FU, so I injected a little bit longer. When her hands started to tremble—not a typical reaction—I took the IV out and called the pharmacy. The pharmacist came up to the unit. She had mixed VP-16 (etoposide; antineoplastic) in the syringe instead of 5-FU. If I had given the entire amount, the patient probably would have died because of the push. I was beside myself. We didn't know what to do. We sweated but tried to be cool about it. We switched the medications around, but we were afraid that the patient was going to infiltrate because the VP-16 was such an irritant. After that, the patient refused additional chemotherapy.

We called the physician to tell him what had happened, and he told the patient. Fortunately, we sort of caught the error. It could have been a big one because the drug was so hazardous. If the patient had a port or a line, she would not have noticed the irritation; she couldn't have felt it. I started to wonder why I hadn't noticed that the drug was a little cloudier than usual and the volume wasn't right. But if a syringe sits ready to use, and if it's red, and if it says 5-FU, 500 milligrams . . .

RITE OF PASSAGE

I was working at a hospital with 34 beds—on a psych unit—and I was maybe 6 months out of school from my basic program. I was usually in charge of this unit, but on this particular night, I was lucky enough to have another nurse. I was on meds. These were stock medications. We used a cafeteria tray and had cards and soufflé cups. Each patient usually came and picked up his or her med, but four patients hadn't. One patient was on nortriptyline; it was a yellow and white capsule. Another patient was on Pronestyl (procainamide hydrochloride), which were two yellow capsules. I picked up what I thought was the nortriptyline, took it into the patient's room, and gave it to her. This patient was a physician; she was depressed and extremely out of it. I gave her the pills and documented that I had given them.

Next, I went to give out the rest of the meds, and there was the nortriptyline sitting there. "OK," I thought, "what did she get?" And then I realized that she had gotten the Pronestyl.

I remember having a very severe stress reaction. It was as if someone had hit me in the stomach: "Oh, my God, this woman is going to die, and it's going to be my fault." I went to the PDR [*Physicians' Desk Reference*] and looked up the drug. Because this patient didn't have a heart problem, I worried about what the Pronestyl does to normal people. Plus, she was on the nortriptyline, which has cardiac effects.

Next, I sought the assistance of the other nurse. There was a doctor on call for the unit, so we called him. He gave us some instructions to monitor her blood pressure, and then he talked to me and said it could happen to anybody. Basically we monitored her blood pressure and gave her supportive care.

We did not fill out an incident report or document the error in any way. I remember that part very clearly. I felt that we had taken care of her, and I was certainly afraid of getting fired. Now I don't know why we didn't document the error. At that time, though, making a mistake seemed much larger than it does now. My own experience has shown me this. But at the time, I remember losing sleep over the error.

I also felt that I shouldn't do this job and should quit—just leave and become a hairdresser or something like that. I realized how easy it was to make a mistake and how it could happen again and again.

I certainly was more careful afterward. That mistake definitely impressed me. It reminded me of getting in a traffic accident; it was that big in my mind. I thought that if I was going to make mistakes like that, I shouldn't be doing this sort of work. I was afraid that something would happen to the patient.

The fact that the patient did not have any major problem as a result of the error didn't matter to me. I thought her confidence in me as a nurse was shaken, and I felt as if I had violated her trust.

I remember that it was a busy night, and I wanted to get these few more meds done. The other nurse on the unit was not very helpful. Most of the time, she was off somewhere else, so I was essentially in charge of the floor.

Right before it happened, I sensed that something wasn't right, but I wasn't sure of what it was. When I became aware of it, my thoughts were, "God, I should have known! I should have picked that up. I should have been more careful." I was in shock and panicky. I thought that I had to do something and felt lucky that I could go to the other nurse; I trusted her, and I didn't feel scared of her.

It never occurred to me not to say anything to anybody. I had to tell somebody, and I told her exactly what happened.

My first questions were, "Is this patient going to die? And what do we need to do?" I really didn't know the meds that well at the time. I thought that something horrible was going to happen and that we had better do something before this lady codes on us.

Now I see the error differently than I did then. It's not that big a deal because I feel more secure. I think that it seemed worse then than it does now.

The medication error was a rite of passage. I think that every nurse goes through something like this. Actually, that's what the other nurse told me. It was almost as if there was an oral tradition; she had made an error and told me what she went through. She consoled me.

Medication errors are going to happen, and they are serious because of the kind of work that we do. It's not like making a typing error, and someone gets the wrong impression from what you type. This is what happens when you make an error in the field of nursing.

The nurse and the physician made the error easier for me. The physician was the best. His compassion, his understanding, and his reality testing in terms of what would or wouldn't happen helped me. He did this without making it OK to make mistakes. He said, "This is serious, but you haven't committed a crime. We will handle this."

What was most difficult for me was the discontinuity between my image of myself—who I thought I was—and who I actually was. Up to that point, I had judged myself as just the perfect nurse. I hadn't made any mistakes.

That error is something that I would like to forget. I prefer not to remember or dwell on it. It certainly wasn't one of the high points of my patient care, and there have been "almost" errors since that one. I salute the patient who says, "I didn't get that green pill today." I'll check.

I think it was the patient's trust that I worried about most. I remember her, can see her, now.

The personal consequence of the medication error was the guilt and my sense of my own competence. Feeling competent is important. I believe that I am likely to make more errors if I am fearful and feel less competent.

For a while afterward, I became really compulsive. The system that we used to give medications was not good because you had to carry the tray with the cart. It was not as if you could go from room to room. It was a psych unit, and you rarely went into the patients' rooms. When you did, you just schlepped the big tray. It wasn't an ideal situation, but that wasn't an excuse either.

We decided, based on the seriousness of the error I made, that reporting it was ethically necessary, regardless of the consequences for me. The patient's welfare was my chief concern.

The error shook me up for a while. I think that the support I received was helpful in resolving it. It would have been much tougher if I had been with someone I didn't trust or if there was a physician working with me I didn't trust. I don't know any more answers to any of that. The circumstances were still those of a tough situation. Seeing the patient afterward was really important. Seeing the patient get better and leave the hospital was also good. She never noticed that I had made the mistake. I was always amazed at that.

There are a number of things to think about. No harm came to the patient; it could have. The people I talked to were supportive. The error was not something that affected my evaluation, although, in retrospect, I feel that would have brought me more closure. I wish the system had been more supportive in terms of documenting an error. Now I know all the reasons why we document med errors.

Now what we're really looking at is seeing the error in the context of the system. The clandestine piece of it is really what stayed with me. I know now that I would have rather reported it. Then it would have been really finished.

I wonder whether other nurses have that experience and don't report it. This isn't a criminal act—an act of negligence. I'm not saying that sometimes it can't be seen that way, but the fact is that these errors are being made. Maybe there is something wrong with the system that we have set up in that it promotes errors. Nurses don't have the space in which to prepare medications; their workload is too much; there isn't enough time. And there are other factors that tend to promote errors. We just have to deal with that. We have hazards in this field that at a building site would never be tolerated.

I've always been appalled at the lack of space that nurses have to prepare medications. That space is a big deal. Granted, it's getting easier, and we have the unit dose now. But I still see nurses with cafeteria trays. I worked in one hospital where the cup didn't fit. The compromises that we have to make when we do something so integral to our work are appalling, and some of the conditions under which we work are almost archaic. One of our nurses one day had to crush a pill, so she picked up the phone and used it. There was no mortar and pestle. That's so typical. We're so innovative that we see everything as having five uses. The phone makes a great pestle.

Summary

Seasoned nurses are in an ideal position to support graduate nurses through their first medication errors. It is important at this stressful time to help the neophyte focus on patient safety, act wisely when monitoring the patient, and document actions taken to resolve problems the patient may have. Just as important is giving guidance to the new nurse, who needs someone to listen and to help him or her move forward from this experience to a renewed sense of professional competence.

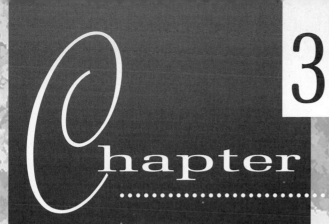

Chapter 3

Making a Medication Error as a Seasoned Nurse

Often when experienced nurses make medication errors, the mistake comes as a surprise. Often they do not entertain the possibility that they will make an error. They are shaken by the episode and question their competence as nurses.

COMPETENT NURSES MAKE MISTAKES

The medication error that comes to mind is fairly recent. It occurred when I was just finishing orientation at the hospital. I was the only RN for 14 very sick patients, and I had two LPNs, which meant that I was responsible for all of the IV medications and some care. It was one of those nights from hell when everything that could go wrong did go wrong. I knew that there was the potential for error, and I kept checking over everything—the meds and the IVs, for example. I had a slew of medications to hang by 6:00, and this one man had a heparin drip.

I can still see it. I noticed at 6:00 that the IV was pretty well finished and I would have to hang up the new bag. The IV tubing was outdated, so I had to hang up the new bag, the new tubing—everything. All of our IV bags are lined up in the medication room. The pharmacy puts them there. The heparin and the aminophylline bags are the same size, and both have red writing across the top, so it's very easy to grab the wrong one. That's what I did.

My error was not caught until halfway through the next shift. I had hung the bag up at 6:00, and they figured it out at 1:00 that afternoon when the patient got back his prothrombin time and partial thrombo-plastin time. They looked at the times and wondered why he wasn't keeping up his prothrombin time. So one nurse went into the room and checked the drip. Now, she should have checked it at 7:00 that morning. She glanced at it and saw what it was. They immediately took the bag down and sent an aminophylline level to the laboratory. His aminophylline level was very low. They called the doctor and told what had happened. Then they hung up a bag of heparin.

When I came on the next day for another 12-hour shift, they said, "Oh, by the way." It was very nicely done. One of the nurses called me aside and said, "Look, this is what happened. It was our fault too. But you hung it at 6:00, and we didn't catch it until 1:00 in the afternoon."

The other nurses treated me well. They decided not to fill out an incident report—maybe because they were going to get in trouble too. But they said they understood how I had made the mistake. Nevertheless, I felt stupid and ashamed. Here I am, with critical care experience from a trauma unit, and I come to this little telemetry unit and I make what I thought was a big error. Their attitude was that it could happen to anybody and I was so busy that making an error was easy.

I was upset about doing harm to the patient, though he didn't have a clue as to what was going on. I was upset about appearing stupid in front of my colleagues. And I was upset with myself.

The only thing I can think of when recalling this error is that I had picked up the bag that said heparin. But then something distracted me, and I put it back down again. When I turned around, I probably picked up the bag next to it, which was aminophylline for somebody else. Now once I pick up that bag, I usually don't let go. You have to pry it out of my hands. Then when I take it to the room, I check it several times—as I'm hanging it up and after I hang it up. I'm insecure.

On that shift when I made the error, all hell was breaking loose. People seem to develop chest pain between 4:00 and 6:00 A.M. We had to go to the ICU to get an EKG machine because the hospital is too damn cheap to get another one. I was the only RN; the LPNs have their designated role, and they will not step over it. They were not licensed to do IVs, and I had a couple that had fallen out. Of course, they all fell out at 5:00 A.M. So I was starting IVs, handing out some oral meds, flushing heparin locks and making sure they were still working, and grabbing the EKG because somebody had chest pains. The dry heparin bag with its old tubing was the straw that broke the camel's back.

When the other nurses told me about the error the next day, I felt so ashamed and so upset. First of all, I pride myself on doing the best for my patients, and that night I almost killed somebody. And I felt so stupid. I was new to that institution and trying to prove myself as worthy of being there in the unit.

Afterward I realized there was nothing I could do about it. I had made a mistake, but it was over and done with. I would have to be careful and learn from it—watch what I was doing in the future and make sure nothing distracted me while hanging up IV bags or giving oral medications.

Later I went to a colleague I trusted—she didn't have a big mouth, and she's an excellent nurse. I told her about the error and that I was very upset, and we talked it over. I also discussed it with the nurse on the unit who had told me about my mistake. She advised me not to worry about it.

Since I made that error, I talk to myself differently. As soon as I found out, it was, "You idiot! How could you do this? How could you be so stupid!" After I calmed down, I told myself, "No use beating yourself over the head. You're human. You probably will make more errors, but let's hope they're little ones. Just learn from it and keep going."

In part, I blame the hospital because that staffing was unsafe. Yet we're penalized for calling up the supervisor and saying we need staff. Anyone who does that is labeled a whiner and doesn't get anything. Also, the hospital wants everything reported! "Oh, report it because we need to keep records for quality assurance, so we can figure out what the problems are and help you." But that's a load of bull. If you report it, then all of a sudden, they want you to retake a medication course or something. It's more punitive. And then you're labeled an idiot.

My peers could have jumped all over me and made life worse, but they were understanding. They told me they've all done it, and I had done my best. The second thing that made it easy was that no harm was done. If, God forbid, that patient had something worse happen to him, I would really be upset! Another reason I didn't get overly fanatical about it was the doctor's attitude. She asked, "How is he? Fine. Oh, don't worry about it."

My opinion of myself as a nurse has dipped, because nurses don't screw up! And I had to work with these people. Would they trust my work? Would they be looking over their shoulders?

You have to deal with yourself. What it is to be a nurse is to do no harm.

One medication error that I reported happened in a critical care setting in a busy trauma unit. It was a phenobarb drip, and again I had a one-to-one patient, with everything going wrong. It was busy, and I had to mix the medication. I remember getting out my calculator and dividing a couple of times. Finally, I put 10 milligrams in the bag. I should have put in 100. Somehow in my calculations, I had left off a zero.

I kept checking the drip because something didn't seem right. I kept going over it, and I kept getting the same calculation.

A couple days later, the assistant nurse manager called me in. Another nurse had found the error and written an incident report. At this hospital, everything had to be documented. They left paper trails all over the place. They insisted on an incident report. So she prepared one, and they just said, "Well, here it is. Just be more careful." End of discussion. But I know that's filed someplace, and if you get too many slips with your name on them, eventually it's good-bye.

Sometimes medications are given incorrectly but on purpose. When I worked at one hospital, I was one RN for 30 medical and surgical patients. I was responsible for giving out oral and IV meds. At this hospital, they gave us a 2-hour leeway. If the med is due at midnight, you can give it at 11:00 P.M. or 1:00 A.M., and it's considered on time. We had 8:00 P.M. meds, 10:00 P.M. meds, and midnight meds. So you know what we did. We gave the 8:00 P.M. and 10:00 P.M. meds together to 15 of the patients, and by then it was 10:00 P.M. And then for the other 15 patients, we gave the 10:00 P.M. and midnight doses together. It was considered routine to give them like this.

I think the administration knew what was going on, but nobody really cared. If they knew you were doing that, they would say not to do it. But it was rampant throughout the institution.

And people need sleep. There's always some physician who writes for meds at 4 A.M. Well, unless they're critical, there's no reason to awaken a patient at 4 A.M. So we would sometimes deliver the tens and twelves at 11:00 P.M. so the patients could sleep. If somebody happened to wake up at 4:00 A.M., we'd give them meds then. Otherwise, we'd wait until 6:00 A.M. That is technically a med error, but it was done throughout the institution.

There's also a lot of confusion when people are off units for tests during the day. A patient would go down to X-ray and might be down there forever. When he came back, he would have missed all his meds.

A LESSON LEARNED:
A PERVASIVE MISTAKE

I didn't realize I had made a medication error. They didn't call me at night, probably because they were so occupied. When I went back to work the next night, I inquired about the patient's health and was told that he had been transferred to an ICU. He had had a severe anaphylactic reaction. I immediately had an anxiety reaction, and my mouth got really dry. I tried to find out what had happened to the patient. By the time the night supervisor got around to getting a report from me, I had found out what had happened. The patient had asked for something for pain, and I actually had followed the order to give him APCs [aspirin, phenacetin, and caffeine]. But the man was also allergic to aspirin, and I hadn't questioned the order as I should have.

The next morning, when the head nurse came on, I gave her my report, and then she had to sit and counsel me about the accident—the incident, as they called it.

I became physically ill too, for two or three days. The emotional impact stayed with me for many days—many months, in fact. What stands out is that I almost killed a patient. It then drove me to the point of exactness. I became compulsive about medications, making sure I was giving the right thing. It was not just five checks or however many checks we had to do. It was not giving medications at all until I knew I was doing the right thing.

I could deal with the blame because I had made a mistake. The part that I couldn't deal with was that people had a tendency to support me by saying that I wasn't used to making errors. They were almost rationalizing my behavior for me, and I didn't want them to do that. I guess I wanted to accept more blame than people felt was necessary. People had a tendency to say, "You shouldn't take it so hard." "You've never done this before, and we know you won't ever do it again." "You're too good a nurse to do this kind of thing." But all I could see was that I was completely responsible for a patient almost dying. I was harder on myself than my co-workers and my superiors were.

I talked to my head nurse—for a long time, because I found her very supportive and very understanding. She helped me realize that I do make mistakes and I'm not infallible. Her calm, accepting manner made it easier for me to go back to work and not feel completely guilty.

I had never made a medication error before, not even as a student, and I couldn't reconcile my action in making the error with my nursing. I guess I thought I was incapable of making that type of error and of not thinking.

I still think about it. It was a stupid mistake, and I was completely at fault. I was too much in the habit of accepting what was written down as the gospel truth and not questioning it. Now I question everything. In fact, I went from being one way to being another way. I started asking too many questions.

After all this time—20 years now—I can see the room; I see the patient's face, know what went on, and remember that the man asked me for something for pain, and I gave it to him. I'm always surprised that this incident has stood out in my mind the way it has. Nothing else has affected me the way that it did. For me, this episode was earth shattering.

WORST CASE SCENARIO

I was in the emergency room on a 12-hour shift at a place where I worked occasionally. There were two other nurses on. I was on triage, and a woman came in with chest pain. She had a pasty look, and her chest pain was dull, so I brought her right back, and she ended up receiving streptokinase [thrombolytic enzyme] from another nurse who was there.

Two nurses prepare the IV drips because it's so detailed. The nurse involved with the patient will keep doing vital signs and start the lines. I became involved in mixing some of the drips, and I mixed heparin. But I had not mixed heparin at that hospital before. The vials were much different from those I was used to; in fact, they had five times the dosage I was used to. So I thought the vial had 5000 units when in fact it was 25,000. The drip and the dosage for the bolus were all calculated at five times more than they should have been. I mixed it up. Then I turned to the nurse beside me and said, "This is what I'm reading." I went over it, and she agreed with me. I never brought that out in the end, because she would have lost her job too. Anyway, I mixed up the drip, and I mixed the bolus. The reason I checked with her was because I'm used to 1 cc being a 5000-unit bolus, and I had 2 ½ cc's in a syringe, so the drip I mixed had 125,000 units instead of 25,000. I mixed it up, put it on a pump, and took the syringe and labeled it with a red label, left it on top of the pump, and told the nurse who was there taking care of the patient. The doctors wanted to hold it temporarily; they didn't want it yet. It was ready and I was leaving.

I went home and went to sleep. Around 6:30 I got a phone call from a very, very nervous nurse. He was asking, "Which vials did you use, and what did they look like? I can't find them, and I think the patient got too much." I got real upset at that, and I told him to look in the trash cans. Then he found them, and he confirmed what had happened, and I said, "Are you sure?"

I was very upset, and I asked for the nursing supervisor. The patient had gone to the ICU. I said, "If this mistake happened, then not only was the bolus a high dose but so was the drip, so please go to the ICU and make sure they shut that off. So she said, "OK." I got dressed and drove down there. First I went to the med room of the emergency room and checked the vials myself. It was clear what had happened.

I went to the ICU to see how the patient was and what the PT/PTT results were running. But since the patient was getting streptokinase, I knew that that doesn't really gauge it because the PT and PTT are out of whack anyway. So I went to the lab and waited for the lab results for the PT/PTT. The patient was not bleeding at that time. I stayed around, and the patient was still not bleeding when I left. The PT/PTT's were still higher than the machine could calculate. I stayed and wrote an incident report that said what had happened up to that point. With another nurse, I calculated what the patient had actually gotten. I looked at what was left in the bottle and confirmed it with the ICU nurse.

There was another error in addition to mine. The nurse who hung the drip made a mistake too. The patient had gotten 100 cc's of this drip, which was five times what it was supposed to be. I calculated what the patient had actually gotten and went to the nursing supervisor. Then I went to the physician who was caring for the patient and told him what the patient had actually received, so he could decide whether to give plasma to reverse the clotting process. Then I called the head nurse of the unit and told her everything.

After I wrote up the incident report and left a copy, I went home. I was due in at 3:00 P.M. again that afternoon, so I slept and then went back to work. I sat down with another nurse to recheck the calculations and saw that the answer was wrong. The numbers were so high, it was difficult to do. We calculated again and came out with a different calculation. I took back my incident report, rewrote it, told the supervisor that was on then, and that was all.

Later that day I got a phone call from the head nurse who asked what happened. When I told her, she said, "Well, I have to tell you that you and the other nurse are being dismissed." I asked, "What's the reason?" I hadn't made errors before. Of course, you never know if you have sometimes, but I don't usually make an error like that. She said that it was requested by the nurse administrator. Then she asked, "When you mixed the dose, did you check with anyone else? If you did, they would lose their job too." Of course, I said no. I don't think any of us should have lost our positions there, so I certainly wouldn't implicate another nurse.

There's more. The patient died. First of all, the patient was having bleeding. What I was trying to determine was, did she die as a result of the error? From what I can gather, it's possible that it was indirect. I don't know. The patient had some bleeding, and she had a history of nose bleeds. We knew that when she came in. That was one contraindication to streptokinase.

The other is that she was 72 or 73 or 75. I forget. Probably she was over the cut-off age for receiving that drug according to the protocol, so she had two contraindications to streptokinase. I don't know if there were any others, but she had bleeding from her nose that wouldn't stop and then they finally gave the plasma to reverse it. They couldn't swan [insert an intra-arterial central line] her because of the bleeding risk. Now I don't know what came first. I didn't read the chart, but it's my understanding that they couldn't swan her because of the bleeding; that may have complicated her care. The plasma may have made her more compromised, into failure, by increasing the work on the heart. Understand, she was an acute MI [myocardial infarction]. She's the type of person who may not have made it with the streptokinase.

My first feeling when this happened and when it came to my attention was that I was sick. I felt like I was sinking. It was awful. [She sobbed.] It will always be upsetting to me because we're always at risk of that. So that was the most impressive part to me. As far as losing my position, I was hurt in a way. But it wasn't that serious because it was a political thing, and I can't take that personally. But it is unusual; it was so drastic. I think that the hospital position was, "Just get rid of this problem. Let's get rid of the nurses."

Now, I think there were some things that I didn't know about. There's a lot they could have done, and I feel removed from the error because I was not there to make any decisions about the patient's care. If I had worked in the ICU and I was still working with her, I would be saying, "Well, I think we should do this or that. Maybe we can manage her better this way," but I was not involved.

After they called me, I was panicky as I left home and went to the hospital. I was hoping it wasn't true. When I started to regroup, I thought, "I have to be responsible about this," and "How can I help the patient at this point?"

The nurses in the emergency room were very supportive; in fact, some of them openly told me about errors they had made. They were very supportive because they knew how upset I was. I talked to them about my concern for the patient and how upset I was that I had made an error.

When I think about that incident, I think about how quickly my career could have been over as a nurse. And I thought about all the time and everything else I had put into my career. Nursing is my career, and I plan to do a lot of nursing. Sometimes I feel vulnerable, and I think that maybe I shouldn't go on. What if I get my doctorate in nursing, and a case comes up and I lose my RN license? What happens to a nurse?

Since making the error, I'm more humble and more cautious. I appreciated the fact that the other nurses shared. You realize that you're human, and you just have to accept we all are; physicians, nurses—we can make errors. This kind of error has a lot of implications. It could harm the patient.

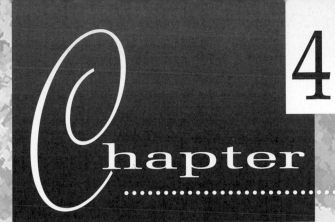

Chapter 4

Nurses' Experiences Making Medication Errors

THE INVESTIGATION

In this investigation of medication errors, a descriptive, phenomeno-logical approach was used to elicit from 16 nurses their personal experiences of making medication errors. The purpose of the study was to describe the meaning of medication errors for nurses. Fifteen of the subjects were interviewed in a private room; one subject was interviewed on the telephone. The interviews, which lasted between 25 and 60 minutes each, were audiotaped and transcribed. Each nurse, who also provided demographic data on a nurse profile form, was asked the following questions:

1. Please try to recall a personal experience that you had when you made a medication error. Try to describe how you felt in that situation.

2. How did the personal experience of making the medication error impress you?

3. What were you trying to accomplish as you gave the medication before you recognized that you made a medication error?

4. What was your experience before making the medication error? during? afterward?

5. If you ever discussed the situation of making the medication error with someone after you realized that you made the error, who was that individual, and what did you discuss? How did you "talk to yourself" or relive the medication error experience after you made the medication error? Describe your recollection of reliving the medication error experience.

6. What differences could you detect within yourself after making the medication error? What made the whole medication error experience easy for you? Difficult for you? Enjoyable for you? Disagreeable for you?

7. Describe the personal consequences of making the medication error.

8. How does your experience of making a medication error that you reported compare to your experience making a medication error that you did not report?

9. Is there anything that you wish to add? Please continue until you

feel that you have discussed your feelings as fully as possible
(Riemen, 1986).

The investigator audiotaped field notes following each interview,
noting general impressions of the subject and the interview itself.

The investigator used the analytic technique of phenomenological
reduction, consisting of empirical description and reflective analysis:

1. Read and reread the transcripts of the descriptions in order to
   gain familiarity with them, acquire a feeling for them, and make
   sense of them. Audiotapes were listened to one to two times and
   transcripts were read two to three times to assist the investigator
   in understanding latent meanings.

2. Extract significant statements specific to the phenomenon in
   order to identify the thematic structures of the experience. List
   thematic structures (categories) and indicators (quotations from
   the transcribed interviews) and organize structures around the
   indicators.

3. Identify and reflect on the meanings of the significant statements
   relevant to the phenomenon for each subject's transcript.

4. Organize the aggregate formulated meaning into a cluster of
   themes to discern a unity of meaning.

5. Validate the clusters of themes by checking whether anything
   contained in the transcriptions is unaccounted for in the clusters.
   The investigator returned to the transcriptions to ensure understanding of meanings and reexamined the written analysis.

6. Reflect on clusters of themes and indicators in order to create a
   description of the nurses' experiences of making medication
   errors.

7. Identify the fundamental structure of the medication error experience.

8. Return to the subjects to determine how the descriptive results
   compare to each subject's experience. Subjects were sent the
   descriptive results by mail and were asked to indicate their agreement or disagreement with the description. A follow-up telephone call was made in order to verify written reactions to the
   description. Changes were integrated into the findings (Colaizzi,
   1978; Knaack, 1984; Stiles, 1988).

MEDICATION ERROR EXPERIENCES: A DESCRIPTION

The investigator organized the common thematic structures of the medication errors by the interviewed nurses into the clusters outlined in Table 4-1 and described in detail in this chapter.

Table 4-1
Thematic Clusters of the Medication Error Experiences

- In Retrospect: Searching for Causes of Errors
- Doing Good and Doing It Right
- Discovering a Medication Error
- Type of Medication
- Nurses' Responses to Errors
- Reporting Medication Errors
- Reactions of Others
- Gauging the Effects of the Medication Error on the Patient
- Relinquishing Perfection: Accepting Human Fallibility and the Possibility of Doing Harm
- The Continuing Recollections
- Reducing the Danger of Error
- Changing Clinical Practice
- Balancing the Good and Bad Effects of the Error

In Retrospect: Searching for Causes of Errors

RNs attributed some of the blame associated with making medication errors to their personal situations at the time of the error. One nurse was a single parent who was obligated to rotate to the night shift, though she slept only briefly (approximately 3 hours) daily. Another nurse made the error immediately before going off duty on a 12-hour shift. A new graduate worked on the evening shift for the first time when she made her first medication error. Another worried about getting off work on time to get a ride home from a relative; the family car had not survived a car accident, and the search for a new car distracted the nurse during the shift. Months to many years later, these nurses continued to review the events surrounding the error to determine whether they could have done anything differently.

Nurses thought that being either too anxious or too secure set them up for the error:

> We do ourselves harm because when you create a level of anxiety that's too high, I think you're more prone to make errors than when you have a level of stress that's a little bit lower that keeps you from making errors. And sometimes I think we've become so anxious as nurses about medications and various other technological things that we focus so much. We somehow make more errors than we would otherwise, and when we do make an error, it becomes a major calamity. We can't forgive ourselves for it.

Fear of making mistakes hovers over many nurses: "It was something that I worried about doing and had all throughout nursing school, and it was during my first job that I made the error." Nurses' fears and self-condemnations may have helped create an error situation.

One RN recalled that nurse administrators pressured her to work overtime, and she ended up caring for unfamiliar patients, including one acutely ill patient, on an unfamiliar unit. She viewed this compliance with staffing demands as setting her up for the medication error that followed. Another staffing situation is too few nurses covering too many patients, as the following comments show:

> It was very busy. Sometimes on nights, I'm sure on every floor, it can be horrible.

> I always felt like if I hadn't been so busy and so pressed, I wouldn't have made such a mistake. Sometimes I feel that we cannot help but make mistakes because we have to take care of umpteen patients and do all these things in 8 hours.

> I had a lot of patients, and one lady had renal failure and a bleeding ulcer, and I was running around doing a million things. I had never dealt with a surgical patient before.

Lack of knowledge about a medication can be a factor. One nurse admitted that rapid development of technology and pharmaceuticals left her humbled and uncertain at times: "It's really dangerous out there. A lot of times you do not have the knowledge base to even think of it."

Nurses cited small-sized lettering, confusing labeling of intravenous medication vials, and unsafe medication distribution systems—including noisy, cluttered conditions and a lack of equipment—as factors contributing to medication errors. One nurse preferred a pharmacy system that sent IV bags to the unit accompanied with the medication to be mixed by the nurse. She thought this system, with the nurse mixing the medication and adding it to the IV rather than with the pharmacist premixing it, was safer.

Nurses made medication errors while working on all types of units: medical and surgical floors, postpartum units, emergency units, medical and surgical intensive care units, and psychiatric units. Often they made the errors when they were nursing students or during the first or second year of professional practice, when their clinical knowledge and experience were limited. Some were afraid to ask questions because they thought they should know everything. They were in a vulnerable period when new nurses get their bearings and become more organized, informed, and efficient. For seasoned nurses, without the vigilance of neophytes, the medication error was more unanticipated and harmful personally and professionally. Moreover, the likelihood of harming the patient was greater, since their lack of vigilance could result in a longer time period elapsing before the error was detected.

In sum, situations become more dangerous when nurses are unfamiliar with patients and with the unit, when they work for agencies, when the number and acuity levels of patients increase, and when new developments exceed their knowledge and expertise. The small-sized lettering and confusing labels of vials of medications add to the complexities of a crisis-laden hospital environment. "Even though they teach you in nursing school to always read something three times over, we could negate all that anyway, because . . . it is just a dangerous, dangerous system. They need to make improvement, especially in those little bottles, those little vials. And a friend said, 'Like what happens if you have one or two days with all the nurses practicing this kind of crazy nursing?' And I thought, you know, he's right." When nurses take on more and more patients, they begin to operate automatically and begin to forget their systems of protection.

Doing Good and Doing It Right

Nurses seek to give medications correctly, even perfectly: "I wanted to give them on time and to make sure that they were to the right person and that it was the right med to the right person at the right time, and to get them all, and not to give them late." Another nurse wanted "everything perfect before I leave." The nurses also used medication administration as an opportunity to teach patients: "I organized my whole day around trying to get it done and talked to patients, and made sure they knew what they were taking, and educate them. And I got them done before 10:30." Many times they attempted to get the job done efficiently and completed the task of giving the routine medications. Other times they had therapeutic intentions; for example, they medicated patients to relieve pain and other symptoms, prepared them for surgery, and kept patients' blood values stable. Since their intentions were for doing good, errors were frustrating and upsetting.

Discovering a Medication Error

At times nurses realized themselves that they had made a medication error: when signing out the administered drug on the medication cardex; when reading an allergy warning in bold print; when making notes in the controlled substance flow record after the medication was given; when seeing the medication that was supposedly given still on the counter; after giving a medication to the wrong patient (who had been sitting on his roommate's bed); or during the narcotics count at the end of the shift.

Other times a nurse discovered a medication error made by another RN. When a nurse realized his error and recognized that the nurse who had mixed the IV medication had also made a calculation error, he called his co-worker, alerting her to her mistake. In another example, a nurse on the day shift saw that a patient's prothrombin time and partial thromboplastin time (indicators of, respectively, coagulation and anticoagulation) were not under control; she checked the IV bag and realized the night shift nurse's error.

When the nurse who made the error realized it, there was an opportunity to keep it private and unreported—for a short time or forever. When there were systems of checks and balances in place, as in the case of the more public narcotics flow record, nurses had greater difficulty hiding the error, and the likelihood that it would remain private decreased. And when another nurse discovered a colleague's error, she could cover up the error if she had compounded it with another mistake or wanted to protect the other RN.

At the time of recognizing that an error had been made, nurses were often in a position to choose to go public or to stay private with their mistake. Also, they felt more in control of the difficult situation as they tried to contain the effects of the mistake. But whether they reported the error themselves or their colleagues reported it, most preferred rapid discovery of the error rather than delayed discovery. It was easier to prevent the harmful effects of the error if time was on their side.

Type of Medication

The most frequent drug error was giving the wrong medication to the patient—for example, gentamicin (an antibiotic) was given IV push instead of a heparin (an anticoagulant) flush, or a preoperative pento-barbital (sedative) was given instead of phenobarbital (sedative). The potential harm to the patient caused by the error was related to the medication, its route of administration and dosage, the time of administration, the organs by which it was excreted, and the clinical condition of the patient.

Nurses' Responses to Errors

Some of the nurses interviewed reacted physically and emotionally when they realized they had made a medication error. Some nurses cried; some sobbed hysterically. Their immediate fear of harming or killing the patient propelled some into a stress reaction with physical symptoms; they described the experience as earth shattering and leaving them feeling upset and nervous, or hot all over. One nurse described a pain burning in her stomach that she readily recalled whenever she remembered the incident.

These anxious and panicked nurses feared the possible personal repercussions of the mistake: of losing their jobs, of lawsuits, of having co-workers who would not trust them, and of facing their own incompetence.

Some were surprised at how dysfunctional they felt. Self-doubt eroded their sense of competence, clinical knowledge, and ability to practice nursing safely. Their pride was damaged, and shame and a sense of inferiority persisted. Nurses cursed themselves, with recriminations that led them to want to hide the error. They directed their anger inward. As their immediate reactions diminished, they felt physically exhausted. They continued to feel guilty, sometimes for many years. Some were depressed and seemed to suffer posttraumatic stress syndrome; they had bad dreams and insomnia following the error. One nurse told of an acquaintance who became suicidal. Some relived the error mentally over and over.

Those who were able to resolve the experience began to recover and eventually were able to put the error into perspective. Nevertheless, many vividly recalled these episodes when similar situations or another nurse's error called them forth.

Most nurses became so immersed in their fear of harming the patient and in the shame and self-recrimination associated with making the mistake that they delayed taking immediate action aimed at dealing with the potential harm that could ensue. They considered not reporting the error:

> *The thing that bothered me the most was that my initial instinct was not to tell anybody because I couldn't imagine what was going to happen.*

> *I didn't want to tell anybody, but I knew I had to. I actually considered not telling because I didn't want to be seen as a stupid nurse.*

Some nurses were immobilized by the fear that they could have killed a patient. Those who acted sought help from others—a nurse preceptor, another nurse, or a physician. Some checked the patient right away. Antidotes did not exist for some medications, but for others, there were other corrective interventions that could reduce harm—for example, stopping the incorrect medication.

Generally when nurses realized that the medication error had been made, they moved through identifiable stages in reaction:

1. Shock: "I didn't do anything, I was just panic stricken."

2. Disbelief: "I got real nervous and real hot. Did I really do that? Did I really do that? How could I do that? It shouldn't have happened to me."

3. Belief: "And when I did realize I did do that, I called my preceptor."

4. Confrontation with the reality of the error: "The first thing I had done was take the guy's blood sugar. It was like 64, or something like that, so I gave him crackers and juice."

If the disbelief stage was prolonged, patient safety might be jeopardized.

Reporting Medication Errors

The nurses interviewed reported the drug error verbally most often. They typically reported the error soon after realizing their mistake and when the next shift of nurses listened to the change-of-shift report. They admitted the error to other nurses, a nursing supervisor, a physician, or anyone else who needed to know. One of the nurses interviewed admitted the error for the first time to the investigator. Some of the errors were shared in postclinical experience conferences and in classrooms in front of fellow nursing students. But no matter what the forum was for reporting, whether verbal or written and whether to neophyte or seasoned nurse, reporting the error provided the nurse with the opportunity to lay the error open to view, to be scrutinized and judged by the group.

Some nurses did have an initial tendency to hide the error. One nurse recalled:

> *It probably didn't take that long, but it seemed like forever before I decided I really had to tell somebody. I knew that I had made, as far as I was concerned, a life-threatening mistake. This was really a horrible thing. How could I cover it up? You really can't cover it up. It's too harmful a thing.*

Another nurse had this to say:

> *You need to have your head ruling more than your emotions. There are instances of emotions versus intelligence. Intelligence sort of wins out in the end, even though your emotions might be strong initially.*

Certainly with every medication error made, a nurse usually considers, even if only briefly, whether to tell.

Most often, nurses considered verbal reporting of the drug error to be sufficient. When they thought that the potential for harm to the patient was high, they made a written report—on the narcotic flow record, the medication cardex, the patient's chart, or an incident report. When the error was discovered after the nurse had left the patient unit, another nurse—the person who discovered the error or was involved in some way in the care of the patient—sometimes wrote the incident report.

Many of the nurses were reluctant to make an incident report and did so only when they gauged the actual or potential harm to the patient to be significant. Some associated incident reports with lawsuits, and some viewed these reports as a kind of punishment, most likely because their mistake was made public.

Incident reports are documents that nurses and other hospital workers use to record events that may result in serious consequences to patients, hospital staff, or the hospital. They need to be used when any situation occurs that is considered by institutional policy to be unto-ward or that staff consider to be worrisome or possibly dangerous. For example, a medication error can threaten a patient's safety and actually harm him. The event should be documented objectively and the report should constitute a factual account of the actual series of events. Frequently medication errors that are reported in incident reports are made part of the nurse's personnel file.

Most nurses were compelled to confess their error and used their reporting of it to clean their slate. One nurse said, "I think that I would have felt better if I had had to make out an incident report. It would have felt kind of like punishment for the crime." Another said, "I just felt that I had to relate what happened, to verify that it had happened." Thus confessing the error often had the effect of making it real, and it provided the nurse with the opportunity to move it to an action stage that was intended to prevent harm to the patient. Most did not like to cover up their errors by not reporting them: "I have a hard time dealing with guilt, and that night, after I got it off my chest and after I started telling everybody, then I just had to deal with what I had done."

These nurses typically looked for a sort of atonement in the form of in-service programs aimed at preventing medication errors or other more formal procedures, such as discussions with the hospital safety com-mittee, to reduce their guilt. "I guess I wanted to accept more blame than people felt was necessary. People had a tendency to say, 'You shouldn't take it so hard.' I was completely responsible for a patient's almost dying, so my own blame of myself was harder than that of my co-workers and my superiors." Those who didn't report the error felt incomplete about putting the error to rest. "That was my own thing to live with. I've never really been able to totally come to grips with what I did. It's always stuck with me that that is what can happen when you don't report, so that's how I keep, at times, sort of reliving it." Con-fessing the error made it real; it provided the nurse with the oppor-tunity to move it to an action stage that prevented harm to the patient.

Not all nurses who made medication errors reported them. In making this decision, they considered the consequences of reporting the error and projected the potential harm to the patient:

I never discussed it with anybody. There was no one in the unit that I was close to. I guess my criterion was that if it didn't hurt, that if it wasn't actually given [an IV medication stopped immediately after the patient complained of pain], I wouldn't report it.

Of course, neophyte nurses have not yet developed clinical judgment, and it is only by discussing the error with seasoned nurses that the newcomers learn more accurately what is reportable or harmful and what is not.

Reactions of Others

Generally the first hospital workers to whom the nurses reported the medication error were other RNs, who typically showered support on the nurse who made the mistake, often reciting their own stories of medication errors in order to comfort:

Everybody else on the floor was wonderful. They all came up and shared their first medication error mistakes and stories. I felt better after that, but it was a few days before I really felt much better. A lot of people talked to me.

The other nurses put themselves at risk by saying, "I gave this and the patient died."

Seasoned nurses were especially sensitive to nurses who had made their first medication error, reassuring them that the error did not mean they were incompetent: "You did the right thing. You went to the right people; you recognized your mistake. That's what makes a great nurse." They also provided good support, outlining ways to deal with the error, appearing to care for the nurse who made the error, and calmly accepting the error. "My preceptor, she's very calming, and very relaxing," recalled one RN. "She says it happens to everybody. It will be alright. We'll take care of it; we'll call the physician." Another advised, "Let's call the surgeons. We'll tell them what happened and see if anything should be done."

Not all other nurses provided support, and some gave bad advice—for example, telling the nurse who had made the error simply to get the correct medication from the pharmacy and give it, or advising altering the records: "Just cross it out and put IV instead of PO [by mouth]."

Physicians reacted to nurse-made medication errors by minimizing them in most cases: "The doctor was really the least concerned. I said,

'I made an error. You ordered an IV medication, and I gave it by mouth.' Then he said, 'Oh, you wanted to change it to by mouth.'" They tended to be protective and understanding and helped nurses deal with the error: "He understood how it happened and helped me deal with it. He made it right in a lot of ways, and that was kind of nice." Some physicians actually changed the medication orders to fit the error. "Oh, no problem," replied one physician. "The guy really did need 100 mg of Demerol rather than 75 mg. I'll just write the order." "They changed the person's medication because I gave them the wrong stuff and it worked." When they anticipated that the patient could be hurt by the error, however, physicians usually reacted negatively.

During the uncertainty following the medication error, both nurses and physicians usually waited nervously to see what the effects of the mistake would be on the patient.

Gauging the Effects of the Medication Error on the Patient

Some patients had no reaction to the medication error. Some died. Death, however, was the least frequent result; moreover, it was usually difficult to lay the cause of death to the medication error alone: "She was an acute MI [myocardial infarction]. She's the type of person who may not have made it with the drug." There were less serious but nonetheless upsetting results—for example, a severe anaphylactic reaction. Sometimes potentially adverse reactions could be headed off by taking appropriate action in a timely manner. The final possible result of a medication error was a beneficial effect on the patient: "It was good for him; it worked. He was more peaceful and in better shape than I had seen him."

As nurses waited for the effects of the error to become clinically recognizable in signs and symptoms, some felt professionally impotent to suggest antidotes or actions that might reduce the harmful effects of the error: "I told my nursing supervisor to go to ICU and make sure they shut that IV off. I felt like I was sinking. It was awful."

Nurses worried about another effect of medication errors: patients' decreased trust in them: "Somehow I had violated her trust and thought that something horrible was going to happen, and we better do something before this lady codes on us. But she never picked up the error." The only patient who was aware of the nurse-made medication error among those interviewed was not upset about it.

Relinquishing Perfection: Accepting Human Fallibility and the Possibility of Doing Harm

Nurses who made medication errors recognized, some for the first time, their human fallibility:

> *And how I got through that was realizing that every human being makes mistakes, and the fact that I'm in health care, dealing with medications and things like that, definitely affects people. Well, it doesn't mean that I'm exempt from making mistakes. Yes, I'm just as careful as I can be, but I'm only human.*

This kind of admission is difficult, since many nurses incorporate into their self-image an unrealistic identification with an ideal, perfect nurse: "I think a lot of us have this innate sense that we have to be perfect all of the time, and every day is not going to be like that. Things are going to happen. That was the hardest thing for me." They acknowledged reluctantly that it is easy to make medication errors and they could do so again:

> *I realized at that point how easy it is to make a mistake—and how it could happen again and again because this is the work we do. This is what happens when you make an error in this field, so I felt as if it was a rite of passage. To that point, I hadn't made any mistakes and had judged myself as a perfect nurse. Certainly there was discontinuity between who I thought I was and who I was.*

Slowly these nurses began to accept the fact that good nurses make mistakes and are not perfect:

> *I was really hysterical. I guess I realized that making mistakes is human, and I am human, so I had to come to grips with the fact that it happened once and could happen again. I needed to bear in mind the chance of its happening again.*

> *After I made the mistake, it helped me realize that in my practice of being a nurse, I would know how to deal with a situation. I realized that making a mistake was not going to mean that I was not a good nurse. I thought for the longest time that because I had made the mistake, I wasn't a good nurse.*

As they recognized that they were subject to human error, they usually resolved to pay meticulous attention to detail and make a commitment to becoming more organized. But they knew mistakes were always a future possibility—as were their consequences, especially that of harming patients: "I cannot get rid of that, the error that I made. What if something happened to the patient? It's my responsibility; it's my error."

As these nurses began to cope with their human shortcomings, they acknowledged the help and advice of seasoned nurses and saw the mistake as something that helped them learn even more about what it means to be a nurse. Additionally, handling the first medication error prepared them for coping the next time an error might occur: "At least I know how to handle it when it comes up, if I do that again. I know that no matter what I do, I'm not going to die. That was about the best thing. I got over it, and now I know if it happens again, I don't have to get that upset ever again." But simultaneously they worried about becoming accustomed to making these sorts of mistakes and feared being cavalier about other errors.

Tied up with the issue of fallibility is the value of doing no harm. For some nurses, this fear was extremely upsetting, even disabling, and it stayed with the nurse until the patient's welfare was assured. For others, it never ended.

When little or no harm resulted, the nurse's relief was palpable: "Total relief. It was like somebody defused the whole situation and let me know that there was nothing that was going to be harmful to the patient."

The Continuing Recollections

It's amazing that after all this time, I can see the room; I can see the patient's face and know just what went on. I remember that the man asked me for something for pain, and I gave it to him. I can remember all the events surrounding it. That's how much of an impact that it made on me. And I have forgotten a lot of things about my personal life.

Even years after making the drug error, nurses could still envision the whole series of events. In their mind's eye, they could still see the medication order's print color and size on the medication cardex, what they were doing as they prepared the medication, and the great emotional impact of the mistake. Some thought that the emotional impact etched the situation in their memories. Some had nightmares.

As they relived and analyzed the experience, they reviewed the events surrounding the error. They tried to note what had caused them to make the error. They reexamined the possibility that they could have killed someone and again felt the physical sensations and emotions associated with these memories. Some perseverated about the error: "I don't think I've ever really gotten over it. I mean it's too fresh in my memory really. It's part of my personality—like something stupid happens, and I mull it over and over and over again, until it's dead." They tended to relive the experience when similar situations arose—for example, when they administered the same medication or when other nurses made medication errors: "Every time there's a staff person on the floor who has a major error like that, you relive it. You relive your own error plus you try and deal with what they went through at the same time."

Recollecting was not always a negative experience. "In my role when I was a supervisor, when people made medication errors and filled out incident reports, I'd tell them how I felt. A lot of times the medication errors haven't been as serious. But every medication error is serious. They feel a little better when they talk to you, and they stop seeing you as the person who just doesn't make any errors whatsoever."

Protection from Error: Reducing the Danger

Nurses have developed different methods of protecting themselves from making medication errors by trying to reduce or even eliminate the risks in this situation. One nurse now checks all medication orders and the labels on the medication three times, as she was taught in nursing school. Another nurse's personal system of protection includes leaving medication in unit-dosage packages in the wrapper and in a medicine cup while carrying it to the patient. Then she checks the medication again when removing the packaging. She uses this opportunity to teach the patient about the medication. A nurse who had made a time-related medication mistake found herself repeatedly checking time: "I look at my watch many times before I give a medication. I usually mark down the times meds are due in red and circle them. I am very focused on the time they are due." Some nurses will not administer medications that are premixed or prepoured by pharmacists or other nurses. One nurse checks with the pharmacy and compares different vials of IV medications. Another has become extremely cautious when preparing medications in vials: "The other thing was being much more careful or recognizing the dangers of working with vials that look alike."

Hospitals develop systems of protection as well. They can, for example, reduce the number of chart forms so that transcription errors are reduced, require the use of controlled substance flow sheets so that these medications can be tracked, and hold quality assurance audits of medication errors. Hospitals continuously work to improve these systems. One nurse said she was impressed "any time I see something that is a significant improvement over the old system. Now when the IVs come out and the pharmacy puts certain antibiotics in them, they don't mix them; they just screw it onto the bag, so you can see what it is you mix."

Clinical judgment refined by experience also serves to protect nurses. In one example, a patient complained of pain in his vein when the nurse was pushing in what she thought was Lasix. She knew that his pain was unusual for that medication and checked the medication, which turned out to be potassium chloride, a drug that could have harmed the patient significantly. Had she not been clinically astute as a result of experience, she might have attributed the complaint to some other problem.

Patients also protect themselves and nurses from medication errors.

Changing Clinical Practice

Nurses tended to check and double-check the medications ritualistically before giving drugs following the error. "It drove me to the point of exactness. I became compulsive about medications, making sure I was giving the right thing. It was not just five checks, or however many checks we had to do. It was not giving medications until I knew I was doing the right thing."

Overall, they were much more cautious, going back to basics or the fundamentals taught by their nursing instructors, and reminding themselves to be more exacting. When in a similar situation to the one in which the error occurred, they mentally stepped back, focused on the work at hand, minimized distractions, and were careful to avoid another mistake: "To this day, whenever I do IVACs [automated intravenous pumps], I step back, and look at the number, and try to make sure that I've put it on the right thing, the right number." They questioned their fit with the job of a nurse and also wondered how the job fit them.

They tended to question everything after the error, especially physicians' orders and the authority of nurse administrators:

I'll fight with anybody, because when they told me to help downstairs, this person had some crazy insulin order, and as far as I was concerned, it was crazy. So I went down to this big shot in administration and said, "I'm not giving it. You want to give it, be my guest." I don't give it, and they can simply go to hell because it makes me think, it's too many close calls.

She added advice through her own slogan: "When in doubt, don't."

Surprisingly, something positive came out of these experiences: "I started asking too many questions. I grew a little more. It was a learning experience."

Balancing the Good and Bad Effects of the Error

For most of these nurses, the experience was made easier by facing the fact that the mistakes were not always as devastating as they imagined. Usually the patient did not die. Additionally, fellow nurses and physicians tended to be understanding and informative, and these reactions helped nurses deal with their shame. Nevertheless, these nurses had difficulty facing the mistake, they often relived the error, and they worried about what their colleagues thought of them: "The knowledge that I might have harmed someone or could have harmed somebody was the most disagreeable, but having to share that with somebody else and wait for their reaction was worse than the reaction itself. The reaction wasn't all bad, and it wasn't all good."

It was not unusual for other nurses and physicians to accept the inevitability of an error. This reaction, though, tended to shake new nurses' idealism: "Surprisingly, another thing that really bothered me was the ease with which it was kind of assimilated into the system; in other words, the attending MD just covered me. And no incident reports. You would probably think that that would make me feel better, because I was off the hook, but it didn't. Actually it made me feel worse."

Nurses worried about what the investigator would think of them when she knew about their mistake. This was especially difficult for nurses who chose not to report a drug error and shared this fact. They did not want to be viewed as bad nurses.

CONCLUSION

All nurses—from recent graduates to seasoned professionals with years of experience—can make medication errors. Some errors are more fateful than others: for the nurse who makes them, for fellow nurses, and for patients. The risks of making these errors can be reduced.

Nurses who administer many IV medications should consistently remind themselves of the rapidity of absorption and effect due to this route. They should assess their ability to focus on the tasks at hand. It may be helpful for nurses who work in high-crisis areas, such as emergency departments and critical care units, to prepare IV drugs for their colleagues to administer, but this is not a good idea. The old rule of not giving to a patient what you do not prepare or pour should still apply.

Often nurse-made medication errors are shared, since the error may go unnoticed by others who repeat the same error. Corporate responsibility needs to be examined, so that the nature of the mistake is scrutinized and future mistakes prevented. Also, if a nurse discovers another's error, the one who made the error needs to be informed of it and supported by colleagues.

Many medication errors go unreported, probably since nurses estimate the harm to the patient as minimal or even nonexistent. Moreover, the shame and pain associated with these mistakes may overrule the nurse's judgment. These practices need to be examined by nurses. Drug errors that are reported are often done verbally rather than in writing. Nurses may hesitate to write reports, feeling that the written record could damage their career. Some view written evidence, especially incident reports, as punishment.

Seasoned and neophyte nurses who make medication errors are typically deeply troubled by their mistakes. Among their fears is the possibility of a lawsuit. Nurses would benefit from an understanding of the legal implications of medication errors.

Nurses need to examine the method by which medication errors are reported. Quality assurance programs may be able to document and track the prevalence of medication errors with increased reporting of errors and more specific and consistent documentation.

NOTES

1. The subjective experience is indispensable in phenomenological studies. Following analysis, the meaning of the phenomenon of making medication errors was explicated (Munhall & Oiler, 1986; Parse, Coyne, & Smith, 1985).

   The credibility of the study was established by the following steps: the subjects were adequately described; the subjects had had the experience of making a medication error and were able to recall it; the data analysis methods were described; the interviews were audiotaped and transcribed; and the subjects verified the results.

2. Following an explanation of the purposes of the investigation, the subjects were asked to sign consent forms that explained the risks and benefits of the study. Subject anonymity was preserved. All interview data were kept confidential. The investigator obtained permission to conduct the study from one hospital's nursing research committee and institutional review board.

Table 4-2
Medication Errors: An Overview

1. **In Retrospect: Searching for the Causes of Errors in Antecedent Conditions and Context**
   - attribution to personal situations
   - administrative pressure
   - medication labeling
   - vulnerable neophytes
   - seasoned nurses and possibility of greater harm
   - degree of vigilance

2. **Doing Good and Doing It Right: Nurses' Intentions When Giving Medications**
   - giving medications correctly, even perfectly
   - opportunity to teach patient
   - therapeutic intentions
   - helping other nurses prepare medications
   - the efficient nurse

3. **Discovering That a Medication Error Was Made**
   - personal discovery
   - other nurses discover

- opportunity to keep error private
- some errors have to be disclosed due to systems of checks and balances
- rapid versus delayed discovery

4. **Medication Involved in the Error**
Potential harm to patient related to
- medication
- route and time of administration
- dose
- organ by which it was excreted
- clinical condition of patient

5. **Personal Response of Nurse to Error**
- crying
- stress reaction
- horror
- fear of repercussions
- dysfunction: self-doubt erodes competence
- self-recrimination
- posttraumatic stress
- paralysis

6. **Reporting Medication Errors**
- verbal and written reporting
- presenting error to peers for scrutiny and clinical judgment
- meaning of verbal and written reporting
- equating incident report with punishment
- personnel file
- overreporting
- confession
- waiting to be punished
- accepted blame
- making the error real

7. **Reactions of Other Nurses and Physicians**
- providing support
- sharing war stories
- providing reassurances
- not supportive—not calling the nurse to inform of error
- sharing responsibility and guilt
- good and bad advice
- physicians minimizing error
- patient harm: nurses and physicians troubled

8. **Gauging the Effects of Medication Error on Patient**
   - death
   - disability
   - beneficial effect
   - no effect
   - undermining of patients' trust in nurses
   - patients unaware of some medication errors

9. **Relinquishing Perfection: Human Fallibility and the Possibility of Doing Harm**
   - fear of harming patient
   - moving past tendency to hide error
   - fear of harming patient disables nurse
   - waiting for the effects of error
   - confronting and accepting human fallibility
   - casting off the ideal, perfect nurse self-image
   - medication error as rite of passage
   - good nurses make mistakes
   - preparation for next error

10. **Nurses' Vivid Recollections**
    - detailed memories
    - repetitive review of events
    - sharing war stories
    - nightmares

11. **Protection from Error: Reducing the Danger**
    - improving labeling of vials
    - reducing patient acuity and nurse/patient ratio
    - three-time check
    - personal rituals
    - clinical judgment
    - listening to patients

12. **Changing Clinical Practice**
    - ritualistic checking
    - stepping back and focusing when similar situation occurs
    - questioning many aspects of role and medication administration
    - sharing stories with other nurses
    - growing from experience

13. **Balancing: Good and Bad Effects of Error**
    - not always life-threatening
    - nurses and physicians supportive
    - worrying about reactions of colleagues
    - personal growth
    - getting off the hook too easily

REFERENCES

Brink, P. J. (1989). Issues in reliability and validity. In J. M. Morse (Ed.), *Qualitative nursing research: A contemporary dialogue* (pp. 149–170). Rockville, MD: Aspen.

Colaizzi, P. F. (1978). Psychological research as the phenomenologist sees it. In R. S. Valle & M. King (Eds.), *Existential-phenomenological alternatives for psychology* (pp. 48–71). New York: Oxford University Press.

Hughes, E. C. (1951). Mistakes at work. *Journal of Economics and Political Science, 17*, 320–327.

Knaack, P. (1984). Phenomenological research. *Western Journal of Nursing Research, 6,* 107–114.

LeCompte, M. D., & Goetz, J. P. (1982). Problems of reliability and validity in ethnographic research. *Review of Educational Research, 52* (1), 31–60.

Lincoln, Y. S., & Guba, E. G. (1985). *Naturalistic inquiry.* Beverly Hills, CA: Sage.

Munhall, P., & Oiler, C. (1986). *Nursing research: A qualitative perspective.* Norwalk, CT: Appleton-Century-Crofts.

Parse, R. R., Coyne, A. B., & Smith, M. J. (1985). *Nursing research: Qualitative methods.* Bowie, MD: Brady Communications.

Riemen, D. J. (1986). The essential structure of a caring interaction: Doing phenomenology. In P. Munhall & C. Oiler (Eds.), *Nursing research: A qualitative perspective.* Norwalk, CT: Appleton-Century-Crofts.

Stiles, M. K. (1988, May). *A phenomenological investigation of the nurse-family spiritual relationship.* Paper presented at the Tenth National Caring Conference, Boca Raton, FL.

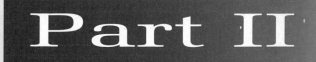

Consensus Building on Medication Errors

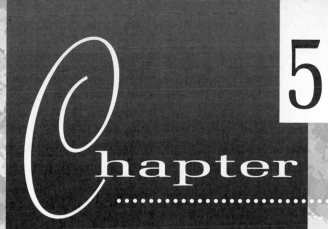

Chapter 5

Group Consensus and Advice

Giving medications is a function that nurses value highly, a theme that becomes clear as nurses consider what tasks remain to them as medication administration is withdrawn temporarily from their clinical repertoire:

> *A lot of nurses feel that giving meds is a really important part of the care that they provide to that patient. And if they're not giving them anymore, then they're not providing that patient care. For a lot of them, it seemed like one of the most important things they did for their patients, and when that was taken away, they were left with just the more mundane tasks, change the bed, etc.*

The knowledge required of nurses in order to give medications is sizable and has been complicated over the years by the demands of the variety of technological equipment used in patient care.

PERFECT WOMEN/PERFECT NURSES: A HOPEFUL ILLUSION

Many nurses view their problems with perfection as tied to the fact that most of them are women: "Some of us have been brought up in our culture with how women are to act, what they're to do in certain circumstances. You see that on nursing units. It has to do with a woman-type reaction." This expectation has generated an ethic of perfectionism. As individuals, nurses expect themselves to be perfect; they do not accept their mistakes or those of other nurses graciously.

Nurses tend to buy into the notion of infallibility: they do not make, and are not expected to make, mistakes. As nurses learn their role, and the boundaries to it, they are trained not to make mistakes: "A lot of our tasks need to be done in a certain way; I was taught to do them in a certain way."

Rigid rules, specified in policy and procedure books and circulated in memos, abound on the topic of medication administration. By following set patterns of behavior, nurses hope to prevent medication errors: "By doing them in a repetitious way, you tend not to make mistakes. When giving meds, you check three times." Nurses thus learn about the inflexible methods designed to prevent medication errors. But they often fail to learn how to adapt flexibly to the realities of the hospital, where events and situations may keep patients from receiving medications in the orderly methods that have been established. For example, a patient may be in the X-ray department and not on the patient unit at the correct time to receive medication.

Nurses gradually learn which aspects of medication administration can be altered. For example, some medications have to be administered according to rigid procedures, but many do not. As nurses gain experience, they see colleagues bend the rules without harmful consequences to patients and begin to bend the rules themselves as they compare the ideal they have been taught with the reality of the hospital and patient care.

DO NO HARM: RESPONSIBILITY FOR PATIENT SAFETY

Doing good for patients and not harming them is an important ethical principle that is made explicit in nurses' education and training. Nursing instructors pass this value on to students in nurse education programs from the start: "The first premise is, 'Do no harm'; that's the first thing you're taught." This professional agenda reflects the fact that medication mistakes can result in the ultimate harm: the death of a patient. "We were taught and we know that a medication error could be lethal. That's what you're taught: it could be lethal." Some nurses, however, believe that nurse educators overemphasize the ever-present likelihood of harming patients while caring for them. Because of this instilled fear, nurses may hesitate to develop alternative and creative methods of working.

The most important reason that nurses report medication errors to their colleagues is that they fear the harm to their patients that can result. They have already accepted the responsibility to care for and about their patients. Being responsible for the safety of patients coexists with being liable when therapeutic intentions go wrong. "When a patient walks into a hospital, we are liable for that person's care. It seems as if when anything happens these days, it's the staff that gets nailed for it." Fears of lawsuits over liability for malpractice reinforce nurses' sense of responsibility. (Most nurses, however, do recognize that physicians are sued more often than they are.)

HOW NURSES REACT TO MAKING MEDICATION ERRORS

Nurses generally move through a variety of emotions when they make a medication error: anger, guilt, frustration, panic, disbelief, and insecurity. Their vigilance increases, and they eventually recognize that they grow as a result of the experience. Hesitating to tell anyone that they made the mistake, they worry about what will happen to them and about their reputation with other nurses.

Losing Control

A nurse who makes a medication error may feel as if she is a failure. The equation is simple: "We have to equate that error with our identity; it stays with you." The mistake is a signal that the nurse is not doing what she is supposed to be doing. Moreover, nurses may permit failure in other people but generally do not allow it in themselves or in other nurses: "Generally, nurses don't say, 'Oh, she made a mistake, she's human.'"

Nurses interpret the events surrounding the medication error and the facts associated with it to mean a loss of control at the individual and unit levels. "I think that most nurses think that when they're on the unit, they are in control of their patients and what happens to them. When they make a med error, somebody else steps in." A nurse who makes a mistake may feel a pervasive sense of loss of control. Someone else takes over responsibility for the patient, at least partially. In fact, nearly everyone working on the patient unit seems to feel a loss of control as a result. Some nurses view a medication error as an indicator of a problem at the unit level: "Maybe the problem is something that is out of your control. Maybe it's something with the unit. I think you should look at it as a symptom of a problem. What does this mean, that this is happening? What are the problems? It might not necessarily be just this person." If the problem that led to the medication error is out of the control of the nurses or not identifiable as an antecedent condition, for example, when a patient is allergic to many medications, nurses must be alert. Their strategies to contain the loss of control at the individual and unit levels have to address the specific nature and history of the events surrounding the error. They stop to analyze the problem and tailor their solutions accordingly.

Perceived Decreased Professional Ability

For seasoned nurses, medication errors may be equated with decreased professional ability. Whether the error is made by an experienced nurse or a neophyte, a pall is cast that has a lasting effect.

Medication-associated mistakes compare dramatically with other sorts of mistakes—say, following a sterile technique incorrectly. "We make errors in other things we do as nurses—treatment errors or procedural errors. We don't look at that the same way we do at medication errors."

Perhaps the correctness or incorrectness of giving medications differs from the degree to which sterile technique is followed. Incident reports are not typically written in the case of violated surgical or medical technique. A nursing student graduates if she or he "didn't quite get the hang of sterile technique, but you did not graduate if you failed your med test or did not know the meds that you were giving your patients." Many hospitals will not hire nurses who do not pass the in-house medication test. A less than perfect grade is an acceptable passing score; nevertheless, perfection is expected when nurses give medications.

Assuming Responsibility

Nurses who do not assume responsibility for making errors may attribute the errors to their situations: "What can I do? I had twelve patients." Other nurses view this sort of rationalization as an indication that the offending nurse does not care for the patient; moreover, they are disturbed by the implications of that response.

Occasionally many individuals are implicated in a single medication error, and they may join together in a cover-up. However, there is no way to cover up an error judged to be serious.

The way nurses react at the time of a mistake can often be attributed to their experience as students. If an instructor treated a student harshly and punitively, putting the person down and raising the specter of killing the patient, the nurse may react to an error as a horrible event. If they could admit the error, go through the process of recording the mistake, and approach it as a learning experience, future events of this nature may not be fraught with so much fear.

It can be hypothesized that the first time a nurse or nursing student makes an error lays the foundation for his or her reaction later:

> It was my first day in the intensive care unit. I made a med error. I could easily have not told my nursing instructor, but I did because I was so afraid that something was going to happen. She was so nice to me because I was almost in tears. Knowing how horrible she was, she was good about it. So if anything would happen later, I wouldn't think twice about saying that I had made a mistake. It's the kind of an experience you've had with your first one that affects how you're going to react to other ones you're going to have.

The manner in which he or she is treated by staff nurses, nurse managers, nursing instructors, and physicians may influence the degree of disclosure this person may make concerning future errors.

DECIDING WHETHER A MISTAKE IS A MISTAKE

What is a medication error in some hospitals or on some units may not be an error for others:

> *It depends on the kind of error and what the perception of an error is on some floors—the meds are an hour late; the meds are not those that they feel need to be given at a certain time; they feel OK about it and just ignore it. At one hospital, they write it up as if it's given on time if it's late, whereas at another hospital, even if it was 30 minutes late, you had to write an incident report.*

Moreover, a physician may be writing additional medication orders that alter the situation, and for a while the decision is suspended: "Going in and getting physicians to change that order may be viewed as an error. But a lot of times . . . I guess that's when they get the order changed, so it's not an error to start with."

SUPPORT FOLLOWING AN ERROR

The medication involved in the error and the type of error made often determine the nature of support that others provide to the nurse who made it. For example, nurses who make several errors involving IV drugs that have potent effects receive limited support. Colleagues who provide comfort and direction take the nurse under their wing and confess their own errors, acknowledging that misery loves company. They may take the distraught offender aside, who often considers leaving nursing, and impress on him or her that others have done the same thing. "My experience has always been that people are very, very supportive, meaning, 'You're upset; you've made a mistake; and you're purging yourself all over the place.' And that's when people usually want to say, 'It's OK; the patient's fine.'" Colleagues who are compassionate try to avoid insensitive remarks that may embarrass the nurse who made the error. At the same time, they want the nurse to realize the mistake and his accountability for it.

Nurses appreciate the support that they receive from trusted friends, nurse managers, or nursing instructors. But unless these others are considered friends, the nurse may not seek their support. Some consider their nurse managers to be very supportive; some do not.

Lack of support for a nurse who makes an error takes different forms. Some nurse colleagues' disappointment clearly shows, and these colleagues may even withdraw from the nurse. Recall that many nurses have high expectations resulting from the message they received in nursing school; nurses do not make mistakes. As a result, they are "very hard" on themselves and others and are "judgmental—some nurses thrive on that." (Seasoned nurses, however, report that compassion seems to be on the increase as compared to the past, when they were new nurses. Now, "There seems to be a lot more leeway in terms of perfection. Twenty years ago they said, 'You've been a nurse for a year. Why don't you have this down pat?'")

Some who recognize the harsher side of these reactions caution against being hard on neophytes who make mistakes: "We should not eat our young." However, responses are frequently qualified by the nature of the mistake: "Depending on what they did, I would not kick them out of the nursing program." Those who are supportive are able to step into another's shoes and agree that they would not wish to be treated severely.

Nurses who are extremely judgmental may be termed predator nurses because they enjoy catching others in their mistakes. These nurses tend to be insecure and attempt to reduce the self-esteem of anyone they catch making an error:

- "It makes them feel better to 'beat up' somebody else who made a medication error."

- "Their reaction could be to destroy you emotionally."

- "One nurse carries incident reports in her pocket, just waiting to fill them out on a nurse—waiting to find something wrong."

REPORTING MEDICATION ERRORS

Some nurses report their medication errors, some do not. They do not report them for various reasons: fear of reproach, of losing their job, of losing their autonomy, of being sued eventually, of making their unit's incidence of errors high for the month. Written reporting adds another task to all of the other work that the nurse is faced with. "You were really busy and you made a mistake, and there's going to be all this stuff that you have to do, and a five-minute report that you have to fill out because you made a mistake." Sometimes other staff nurses encourage the nurse not to report the error. And permanent nursing staff say that agency nurses tend not to report medication errors since they may not return to that hospital in the future.

Whether nurses report medication errors relates to their estimation of the seriousness of the harm that may result: "If you know it's going to cause a problem for a patient, then you report it." But if it appears that nothing will happen to the patient and no clinical effects are observed, the nurse may not report it.

When nurses report an error, they seek support from colleagues, reassurance that the patient will be unharmed, and confirmation they are not the only one who has ever made this kind of mistake. Reporting is a type of confession and relieves the nurse of a burden that could remain buried for a long time. A few seek a middle-of-the-road approach to handling the error, where a "hide the problem" solution is balanced with "I'm going to get you and tell the world." They share the error with their colleagues or the nurse manager.

Putting the medication error in writing makes it real and permanent and impresses the nurse with the fact that she made a mistake. Through a written admission, the nurse who made the error takes on the responsibility for it. Moreover, the report is permanent. The kind of error made can be analyzed in an attempt to prevent future errors of the same nature. Nurses prefer writing incident reports on their own personal errors, since they fear being "hung" by another nurse or by a physician.

The negative aspects of writing incident reports, however, far outweigh the positive aspects. First, writing the incident report is thought to release the hospital from liability for the mistake, with the onus on the individual nurse. Some years later, the incident report could come back to haunt the nurse, a frightening prospect: "Nurses realize that there are legal issues that are tremendous. I think that nurses are really concerned about malpractice."

Incident reports become part of the nurse's permanent record and theoretically follow the nurse during the course of her or his career. Moreover, they are not always held in confidence (although they should be); nurses report that they are often left lying around or are even posted on the walls of nursing units for all to view.

Not all nurses understand the legal consequences of incident reports, however. Lawyers suggest that the nurse detail the error in the patient's chart but not record that an incident report was completed: "Let the lawyer figure that out." In some hospitals, policy requires a written incident report. In this case, a patient's lawyer will feel compelled to look for it. One final piece of nursing advice is that "the legal strategy is to wait as long as you can before going back, so everybody's memories will be extra dim." If the incident report is discovered, it serves as one of the only records detailing the error.

From the Command Post: Responses of Nurse Managers and Administrators

Nurse managers and administrators agree that there is not a wide margin for error in nursing; the human consequences of nurses' errors can be death. This sobering realization helps to explain nurses' extreme reactions to mistakes of this sort.

Nurse managers notice that fellow staff nurses withdraw their presence, and therefore their support, from a nurse who makes an error. Often there is no face-to-face condemnation. Rather, the level of support changes, and the other nurses attempt to overcompensate for the area that they determine the nurse's weakness to be. They converse among themselves, discussing the other nurse's carelessness. Mistrust spreads.

The way in which nurse managers deal with the nurse who made the error depends on individual managerial style. At one extreme is the manager who would bring it to your attention, and she would talk to you. She's understanding. At the other end is the nurse manager who would bring not just medication errors but any incident up at the nurses' station where everyone could hear her.

A medication error alerts the manager to a problem and may create doubt in her mind about the nurse. The reaction depends on how many times this has happened. The situation and the drug dictate the response.

Nurse managers should counsel their staff following the error. They recognize most nurses' need to admit their mistakes: "A lot of times nobody but the nurse knows it and has to just 'fess up' because they're afraid of the implications it would have with the patient. Nurses in general are tempted to tattle on themselves with great freedom." Depending "on the amount and the seriousness of the error," it may be written in the nurse's record, where it stays.

The harshest kind of discipline next to suspension and firing is a written incident report, with the subsequent obligation on the part of the nurse manager to write the event up for the employee's record. Nurse managers are aware that the incident report results in a permanent notation on the employee's record: "It's a severe discipline issue—something that is going to be on the record somewhere." Although incident reports are not supposed to be linked to discipline, if a nurse is implicated in such a report, "minimally you're going to get talked to, so it's an unsaid little rule that at least you're going to have to have a discussion with somebody in authority."

Incident reports can have a judgmental cast to them. Nurses' and physicians' comments on them can be derogatory to the offending nurse. When this happens, the report loses its objectivity and becomes a mechanism for attack. At this point, a vigilant nurse administrator steps in and asks for an objective rewriting of the report.

Additionally, public scrutiny of the error is ensured when an incident report is filled out: "You're really in your underwear up there."

Nurse managers see the systems problems that accompany medication errors and acknowledge that no one is infallible. They see their nurses in the middle—a link in the human chain of medication errors along with pharmacists and physicians. If someone else makes a mistake that leads to an error, the nurse may not be able to stop or even control the events associated with it. This leads to frustration and anger: "I did what I was supposed to, like I checked for times, and then I made the mistake of trusting those other people to do it right too."

Compared to nurse managers and directors of nursing, a chief nurse executive may take a hard-line approach to medication errors, specifying no errors as the only acceptable standard of practice. Some attribute errors to nurses' not following procedure. Procedure, in this case, exists as a protective device to ensure that no errors will occur if medication procedures and policies are followed as written:

> *I'd like to suggest that we're soft peddling a lot of this. And I think carelessness is related to this. There's a lack of compliance with the established procedure. A whole lot of times I see that nurses have not been as thorough, when every time we ask, "Well, how in the hell could this happen?" There's a lack of thoroughness in conforming to the rigidity that must take place in this case, because we have to approach zero defects in this; a patient's life could depend on it. Our responsibility is to guarantee them a safe level of caring.*

This chief nurse executive was not alone in the fear that nurses will consider errors inevitable: "My big fear is that we can't do anything about it—'Everybody makes that error'. I don't want that to happen."

Nurse managers, directors of nursing, and chief nurse executives are privy to the big picture at the unit, cost center, and department levels. They see how nursing fits in with the larger hospital system. They are aware that few hospitals collect data on nurses who make medication errors, as well as detailed descriptions of errors that are reported. They know that they and their nurses are doing well, so that not many changes in policy are instituted: "The numbers at the institutional level would suggest that we're always doing better than baseline. Therefore, there's not the push to make it better because we show continuous improvement. We think improvement is largely a product of awareness—confronting people who have made errors." Some of them resist describing nurse errors in detail:

> I just experienced this big, huge medication error. The doc, who was essentially the person responsible for initiating the error, wrote this horrible dosage. And the nurse didn't pick up on it and gave it. But the nurse's fingernails were pulled out, and she's fearful of the discipline. But the doc just said, "Calculated it wrong; rewrite the order." So there's a difference in how people own it too. As much as I think it would be nice to quantify different nurses' abilities and medication errors, there's just something that irks me about it.

The tempo of a patient unit influences the incidence of medication errors. According to one nurse manager, the way her staff perceives the pressures of the unit determines whether they see themselves as able to follow the procedures associated with medication administration. Staff need to feel that they are supported so that "they can slow down and look at all the things they're supposed to do." On the other hand, a unit that has the temporary luxury of a slower pace may experience more medication errors. Nurse managers think that staff need to feel a certain tension in order to perform well: "On those easy days, your adrenaline isn't carrying you, so you don't have that little extra push to keep you at your peak. Nurses aren't used to having the luxury of doing things at a very slow, easy pace."

When an error takes place, the nurse manager does not minimize it and may focus on how to prevent the same series of events from happening in the future. Listening to the nurse is important. Inexperienced nurses and nurses new to the hospital or the unit need a lot of support. Experienced nurses are especially devastated when they make an error and may need more support than the others. In many cases, the nurse manager sees that the nurse who made the error is extremely sensitive to colleagues' comments: "You have your wound on your sleeve now that you made the medication error."

The ways in which individual nurse managers deal with their staff depend on their personality and what they bring to the situation. Most nurses are very hard on themselves and upset about the mistake. "They're attempting to own what happened, and they're really beating themselves up more than I could ever 'beat' them." The nurse manager validates what the nurse did incorrectly and helps to move the nurse past this difficult point. They note, regrettably, that nurses may equate their career with this one error. They accentuate the positive aspects of the nurse's performance as they discuss the behavior that led to the error. Some may find it difficult to discipline a fellow professional: "I feel very awkward saying, 'Here's a discipline document because you've made a mistake,' when I could make that error too."

The extent of discipline depends on the error and its consequences and on the reaction of the nurse:

> *A lot of it hinges on how the nurse responds to the error. If the nurse takes ownership for the error, any discipline you give is nothing compared to what they've done to themselves. But when I see a nurse who tries to blame someone for the error, or acts like, "So what's the big deal? Nobody died," then I tend to be stronger with a formal discipline.*

Nurse managers discipline their staff in various ways beyond a formal meeting and documenting the error in the nurse's personnel file. They may require homework by the nurse, such as reading articles or completing a posttest after following a self-instructional module. The nurse manager may suggest that the nurse be especially attentive to her or his preceptee, teaching the details about and technique of giving the medication that was involved in the error. They involve the nurse as much as possible in rectifying the error, while noting the pain that lingers following the error experience.

Nurse managers put the pain of the staff member on the back burner and worry about the consequences of the error for the patient: "You look at the patient, evaluate the outcome, and do whatever you need to do to make sure that it's fixed." Next, they notify risk management personnel to ensure that liability for the error is clear from the beginning of the incident.

Nurse administrators argue implicitly that it is a privilege to practice nursing. Because of this privilege, nurses must monitor themselves and others so that patients receive safe care:

> *The patient's right to be ensured safe care takes precedence over the nurse's ability to make mistakes. We should do all these things to save the nurse and to make sure that they understand that they're a valuable nurse despite the error. But I am also concerned with developing a milieu in which it's overly tolerated to the point that it becomes an acceptable level of performance. I think the patient's right to safe care precedes all of that, all of our rights to make mistakes.*

Physicians' Responses

Physicians display various responses to medication errors as well. Often they tend to minimize the error, changing the chart to fit the nurse's mistake so that it, in effect, disappears from the record. "You call the physician, and the physician says, 'Oh, it's no big deal.' They help you with your rationalization, and they feed into that mind-set." (Some nurses think that other nurses should be this supportive.)

Other physicians may be rigid about their orders, and certainly they have every right to refuse to change the order as written. Even if a nurse tries to influence a change in the written order "because I gave this med early," the physician may hold firm. This decision is influenced by many factors, including the medication and its intended therapeutic effect, as well as the physician's personality and the fact that the physician may resent the request. "I've heard nurses who call doctors and say, 'I made an error,' whether in time or dosage. And doctors get all mad, and they say, 'What am I supposed to do? Give you an order for something I never wanted to be given?'" A nurse in this situation, because of the stress associated with the medication error, may not see that the requirements of certain medications—their action, dosage, and timing—may stop the physician from acceding to the nurse's request. At this point, the nurse might recognize the power of medicine and nursing and seek a solution to the consequences of the mistake by retaining a lawyer, for example. "Nursing is still an oppressed group. We don't believe we have power, and we're dealing with a very powerful infrastructure."

THE PUBLIC GAUNTLET AND THE SCARLET LETTER: THE PUBLIC NATURE OF MEDICATION ERRORS

Verbally reporting an error makes it public, as do the discussions that follow as shifts change and nurse managers and their assistants track the error like detectives. Generally, however, the account is limited to the nursing staff assigned to the patient unit, the nurse managers at monthly management meetings, the administrators in the department of nursing service, and the physician to whom it was reported. The patient may not know of its occurrence unless "you go running in there and you can see the pill on their lip—and you yell, 'Don't swallow that!'"

The incident report, because of its permanent nature, serves to attach the offending nurse's name to the mistake for years and makes a major error available to a larger public, including the quality assurance director, the hospital risk manager, and lawyers. For this reason, nurses view incident reports as "horrible." And to make matters worse, some units ensure the public confession by placing the report in a prominent place:

- "You post it on the nurses' station like a Christmas tree ornament."

- "You take the incident report, with your name on it, your sin, and it gets taped either on the desk near the monitors—honest to God—or on the front board where the assignments are. Right there."

- "I used to know a head nurse who posted it. I really thought she was doing it so that everybody could see it. If you were on it, you wanted to throw it in the trash, and some people did."

HOSPITAL MONITORING

Quality assurance monitoring tracks medication errors on a patient unit and hospital-wide basis. Units set percentages as targets to aim for in order to eliminate medication errors. Some set targets of 100%, meaning that no medication errors should be made; this perfect, error-free target is seldom, if ever, achieved. A target influences the reporting of medication errors: "Certainly your unit doesn't want to be the one that has the highest number of medication errors. People will say they gave a med at 12:30 when in fact they gave it at 2:30." Some hospitals have posted these targets and the percentages actually achieved on each unit's bulletin board. "For the most part they were always in the 90s, and we would see who was going to have the highest percentage in the hospital." Recently, this practice has stopped in this hospital: "They haven't posted this in a while, but it was a big thing. I don't think they like to do it just to show the doctors that the nurses are doing something wrong."

Some hospitals are developing and using point systems to assign scores to employee errors, and disciplinary actions may be based on these scores. Similar to the incident report, this record of points stays in the nurse's personnel file and follows the nurse. Many nurses are unaware of these point systems. But those who are react negatively: "You get points for having made a med error . . . a demerit system. Do you stay after school or what?" Nurse administrators, however, view these systems as a way to track errors and carefully counsel nurses who make errors.

SHARING WAR STORIES

The topic of medication errors taps nurses' memories of past errors they and colleagues have made. These stories are instructive and serve to socialize nurses into the ways of the profession. They help the nurse who made the error confess again the mistake, which she or he is unable to forget totally. Also, by relating worst–case scenarios of how they and other nurses have had the same sort of experience gives comfort to others. Thus, these war stories serve to support the nurse who recently made a mistake.

"The patient was harmed . . . "

She was giving Valium, IV push into a hand, and we both watched the lady's hand turn black. Talk about somebody who was scared to death of being sued! As it happened, the patient died in a couple of weeks. The lady never regained circulation in her hand. That was 15 years ago.

I know a patient who died because of potassium chloride. They used to come in a brown ampule that looked like another drug.

"Because I have clinical knowledge . . . "

I was working as a nurse practitioner, and one of the patients had an asthma attack. I ordered epinephrine for the patient, and I had the nurse come in to give the epi. She had misplaced the decimal point on what my order was and had twice the amount of epi she was supposed to have. She started to inject it, and I looked at her. I was standing there with the patient, and I looked at her syringe, and I knew that she had twice the epinephrine that she should. It looked like it was full. I knew she had too much. I don't know why I never said anything to her; I didn't want to alarm the nurse. She had the needle in this patient's arm; it was an infant. She didn't inject it. She just sat there, and she looked at me and just froze. She walked out of the room upset. There was a lot of tension because the child was in a lot of respiratory distress. She picked up on my body language, that I was just about to die.

"Someone has to be punished . . . "

The head nurse had decided that because only one or two nurses were making errors, she was going to punish everybody on the floor. She assigned one nurse to be the med nurse for all the patients and took away giving meds from all the other nurses. It created an unbelievable, horrible situation on the floor. It was very difficult to bring students into the situation. You felt like everybody was being punished, and it was just really a bad situation.

An LPN allowed 1000 cc's of fluid to run in for 15 or 20 minutes, so I took her aside and reprimanded her for this. I explained it to her and asked her if she understood the ramifications of this error. And I was the one who was put on the carpet, because it was a unionized hospital, and I didn't have a union representative there with me. She got off scot-free, and I was the one who was put in hot water.

"We join together to survive . . . "

One of the residents had written orders, and the nurse had followed through on them. And then he took the orders out of their chart. Somebody saw that he threw them in the trash. So the nurse administrator was brought in about that. We found it balled up at the bottom of the trash can. We had to show it to the administrator. That was the only time I saw the administrator involved. That was frightening.

"I worry about the chemically dependent nurse . . . "

We caught someone with a tourniquet around her arm, and the count was down two Demerol. And she was in a room with the door shut, but because we didn't see her inject it, they couldn't do anything. It was horrible. You had to have someone go with you to get medication, to the narcotic cabinet, and watch her sign it.

These two girls were drug buddies. They always worked the same shift. They were covering for each other.

"This error happened because . . . "

She was busy double shifting. She was doing overtime. Some of our patients are really long term. I was a supervisor. Someone gave the patient lidocaine and shouldn't have given the patient lidocaine. The patient went into complete heart block and needed a temporary pacemaker. This nurse was continuously given overtime. She was literally too tired to recognize the difference between the medications.

STRATEGIES TO REDUCE MEDICATION ERRORS

Nurses blame medication errors on many causes—for example:

- The demands of a busy unit.

- Changes in vendors that supply medications to the hospital with associated changes in medication packaging.

- Clinical knowledge that is shared by a few and not formalized in writing so that all nurses who care for patients requiring those drugs can benefit from the information.

The system of medication administration used affects the rate of medication errors. In the past, cards and silver trays with insert holes for soufflé cups were common. Modern administration systems—unit dose medications stocked in patients' rooms and computerized systems that dispense controlled drugs, similar to a money access machine—generally have reduced but not totally eliminated medication errors: "The computers were down, and a patient was being transferred off my unit. The orders were written, but the nurse on the floor never got the orders. They never showed up anywhere, because they were computer orders." Certainly this type of problem and others do occur; nevertheless, computers have improved the prescription, dispensing, and administration phases of medication administration. Calculators are also indispensable in performing drug calculations.

Nurses notice a pattern of medication errors: "In the summertime, not only do you have new interns and residents, but you have an influx of new graduates. There's nothing scarier than an intern and a brand-new nurse." Experienced pharmacists and nurses, however, help new personnel gain useful information related to medications and their administration. Sage patients also help nurses avoid errors: "Even when I'm sure, if the patient says anything, I go right back and check it."

Some of nurses' socialization is aimed at reducing errors. Preceptors and instructors teach new nurses to question new orders and the reasons patients are receiving certain medications. Experienced nurses stimulate others to question things, especially if they notice a lack of curiosity during change-of-shift report. "I always say, 'Look at what you are giving and why you are giving it.'" When a new nurse makes an error, the experienced nurse takes the neophyte to task and demands a review of the situation: "She was distraught about the whole thing, and I was too. She made a mistake, and so you talk about it and what you can do to keep it from happening again."

PROFESSIONAL PRACTICE

Most of the time, nurses regulate their practice in relation to medication errors at the level of the patient unit. Unless it becomes a major issue, the error is fairly anonymous above that level. This highlights the fact that nurses often function autonomously as they care for patients. They use their clinical judgment to decide, for example, whether "this patient needs more med now, since I can't wait 6 hours to give another dose." This is the time that they seek the physician or act on their own in response to the situation.

Ideally, nurses who make a medication error follow the standards of the profession and uphold the value of avoiding harm to the patient. That may be why they prefer to oversee and take responsibility for their own professional behavior. Writing the incident report allows them to own up to the mistake and to retain some control over the situation. The reaction of the individual nurse manager can help or hinder the nurse at this point: "If they know that their fingernails were pulled out because they made this med error, they're going to be bonkers trying to make out their own incident report. Depending on how their nurse manager deals with the incident report will make their reaction different."

Summary

- Provide periodic inservice education programs on new medications.

- Test each nurse's dosage calculation skills yearly.

- Revise procedures for medication administration to allow for flexible times of administration for medications that do not require specific times of dosing.

- Realize that a medication error signals a problem for a nurse or other hospital employee or for the systems of prescription, transcription, dispensing, or administration.

- Realize that a cluster of medication errors signals a potentially greater problem at the unit or nursing service organization level and is worthy of rapid responses by nurse mangers and clinical directors.

- Analyze the events preceding and accompanying medication errors; tailor solutions to the details of the problem.

- Encourage more open reporting of medication errors with an emphasis on solving problems at the level of systems through quality assurance approaches.

- Support nurses who make medication errors.

- Let staff nurses know that medication errors are serious, and alert all nurses to systems problems.

- Approach medication errors as opportunities for nurses to learn and grow.

- Maintain open communication with physicians and pharmacists.

- Encourage nurses to seek trusted advisers to tell their medication error stories to.

- Help predator nurses change their approach to one of a quality assurance focus.

- Invite a hospital lawyer to provide a yearly inservice education program on incident reports and personal and hospital liability issues.

- Hold incident reports in confidence.

- Give staff nurses permission to slow down and focus on the job at hand when administering medications.

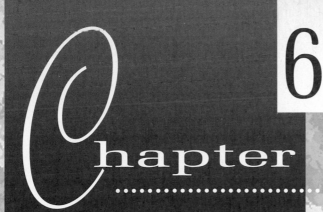

$\mathcal{C}$hapter 6

Quality Assurance Directors and Risk Managers: From the Outside Looking In

QUALITY ASSURANCE DIRECTORS

Quality assurance (QA) directors for nursing are responsible for monitoring the safety of nursing care in hospitals. More often than not, they are involved in situations in which nurses make medication errors.

A QA nurse investigating a nurse-made medication error focuses on the legal consequences of the error rather than on its personal consequences. (She may personally identify with the nurse who made a medication error but as a rule does not personally contact the nurse. However, QA nurses admit that they are aware of the complexities and distractions associated with medication administration and seek to protect other nurses.) This person analyzes how the nurse and the department of nursing could have prevented the error, and searches for a trend or pattern in an attempt to see whether the error fits into a larger picture. Perhaps the nurse who made the error had made several others previously, or perhaps many nurses working on that patient unit have made errors. They are studied as part of an aggregate in relation to the whole department of nursing. Specifically, the QA nurse compares error trends in part-time and full-time staff, RN and LPN, time of day and shift when the error was made, and type of error. These patterns are examined over 1-month, 4-month, 6-month, 9-month, and 12-month time frames. QA nurses repeatedly ask themselves what any trends mean.

QA nurses search for systems problems that lead to medication errors, hoping that the nurse involved in any errors is not culpable. They seek actions aimed at preventing future mistakes. The explanations or theories of the errors that they construct are offered to multidisciplinary committees in the hospital, such as the pharmacy and therapeutics committee, and outside the hospital to the state department of health. These explanations are also scrutinized by the attorneys for the hospital and later by attorneys representing families considering legal action. QA nurses do not meet the family members face to face. The medication error situation remains at an impersonal level.

When an error is discovered, the QA nurse asks the following questions:

- Was the medication error reported?
- When was the error reported?
- Was the system responsible for the error?
- Was the nurse responsible for the error?

- Does the record of the involved nurse reveal a pattern of errors?
- Is this medication error part of a larger trend?

The QA nurse next asks if the right people know what happened. Often even the nursing staff who work on the same unit during different shifts may not be aware of the error. Their notification, however, is not so important as are communications with the staff of the legal department, the administrative staff within the department of nursing, and the quality assurance staff.

As QA nurses go about their job, they consciously contain the facts related to the medication error. They investigate carefully and systematically, with all intentions of reducing rumors. Their fact-seeking mission uses interview techniques to gather information to describe the events associated with the error. Next, they evaluate the incident report of the error; they want just the facts recorded on this document. They weigh these facts against the facts included in other documents, once again affirming their desire to keep the error contained. In sum, the crisis containment approach of QA nurses is aimed at gathering facts, containing the error, resolving the error, and encouraging hospital staff to report errors but not dramatize them. These nurses consider themselves to be members of the fellowship of nursing and are dedicated to protecting the nursing department. They are searching for systems, not human, errors.

When rumors threaten fact, more discussion may be warranted. In this situation, QA nurses persuade those in the rumor mill to consider the nurse who was involved, since "bad things happen to good people." Moreover, the nurse who gossips may have been the person who made the error and fears being fired.

QA nurses recognize the emotional consequences of the medication error for involved nurses but are concerned primarily with the immediate effects of the error on the patient's welfare, the extent to which the error will influence subsequent care, medications, and the likelihood of another error. They work with nurse managers and directors of nursing, who have a great ability to influence changes designed to eliminate system problems. Nurse managers also add another perspective to the error. Together the nurse manager and QA nurse discuss what happened when the error occurred and plan to minimize harm to the patient. They are especially interested in gathering all of the facts, since the nurse involved in the error may not report all the facts immediately. Also, they propose solutions to eliminate future errors. Additionally, pharmacists and risk managers offer advice and strategies. Pharmacists offer knowledge of the effects of medication errors, and risk managers the liability issues. QA nurses change their approach to individuals involved in the error, depending on their role in managing the mistake and the nature of the mistake.

QA coordinators find it difficult initially to be removed from day-to-day events and people in the hospital. They are insiders and outsiders. They have most likely made medication errors themselves, and most surely identify with each nurse's error; however, they shuttle back and forth from the immediacy of the clinical area to the more distant analysis of events on the unit. They try to understand the medication error in the light of what else was happening on the unit. They remain sensitive to the nursing staff, but their objectivity and separateness from the staff and the unit help them to see the whole picture more objectively.

They may find it difficult to balance objectivity with sensitivity, and may also find it difficult that after a medication error occurs, "there is nothing that you can do." Another source of frustration lies in conflicts that become apparent as different managers analyze medication errors and arrive at different and conflicting solutions: "Your suggestions may not make sense, even though you know it will change the outcome and prevent something from happening."

Often nurse managers and QA coordinators are in conflict because the QA nurse encourages the nurse manager to analyze the medication error more objectively. It is difficult to confront negative information about the systems and personnel of a nursing unit. Furthermore, a lot of nurses who are regular staff blame mistakes on per diem staff. But QA nurses know that statistics indicate that regularly scheduled staff make most of the medication errors.

QA nurses as a rule enjoy seeing their plans implemented and hope they prevent medication errors. "You know that you can prevent it in the future. You could prevent trauma to a patient, a nurse, and the institution." They understand that accidents and errors stimulate creative outcomes, and they know that they can analyze people and systems.

Incident Reports

Incident reports are important to QA nurses. These reports often contain details about the events of the medication error—sometimes enough data for trend analysis.

Staff nurses, however, dislike incident reports: "The form itself is sort of a negative item. The nurse has made a mistake, has to fill it out, has to hand it to an authority person—a nurse manager or a supervisor—and the QA coordinator is going to come back with it. They don't really ever want to see it."

Incident reports have a bad reputation. Hospital staff, including nurses and physicians, may fill out an incident report to punish another clinician. Also, an incident report is never made out for a positive event, so it is always viewed negatively. Some hospitals have changed the name of the document to adverse event report; nevertheless, the report still makes the medication error visible and public, and its stigma therefore remains.

QA coordinators view incident reports as nursing's private business since they involve nurses' mistakes. They use their leverage as QA coordinators to protect the confidentiality of patient, nurse, unit, and department. At the same time that they look out for the involved parties, the coordinators lament that there is no wrap-up in the form of a support service for the nurses or pharmacists involved in medication errors: "We don't talk about how anybody felt about the whole process." They consider a medication error to be similar to a fire in the hospital. After such a crisis, there is a debriefing of the employees who were involved. A medication error calls for crisis intervention.

Sharing Medication Error Statistics

Hospitals calculate their own medication error statistics but do not share these numbers with many who work in the institution, nor do they compare these numbers with those of other hospitals. The pharmacy and therapeutics committee, traditionally chaired by a physician, focuses on error statistics but usually does not examine the number of errors in relation to the number of medications prescribed, dispensed, and administered. Nor do many hospitals have computer systems that document these numbers. Some pharmacies count the number of drugs dispensed, so error rates could be calculated, except that this calculation would not be a true reflection of actual medications given since it would not include as-needed medications. In addition, the number and types of personnel involved in medication administration add to the complexity. Hospital insurance carriers possess information about the patterns of medication errors and other hospital problems but do not share this information.

QA nurses wish that this information were widely available. They could use, say, a composite profile of hospitals' error rates to develop plans designed to reduce and eliminate errors. Profiles of individual employees and their mistakes at work could be employed to develop educational programs to support individual employees and to reduce their rate of mistakes. "Management's and administration's responsibility," notes one QA nurse, "is to support the workers, to retain them, and to make sure that the mistakes are included in workers' employment counseling." An employee with a high error rate could be counseled to apply for a position that does not include medication administration. Patient safety is always an issue for QA coordinators.

The Big Picture

Unexpected factors may come to light during QA coordinators' investigations of medication errors. For example, the nurse may be dyslexic or the medical clerk may need new glasses. These issues are often dealt with by the QA coordinator on a one-to-one basis, although always with an eye on the big picture in the hospital: improving the quality of patient care services.

The QA coordinator sees larger patterns in the delivery of care than does the nurse manager, for example, who is unit based in scope. Because of the wider view, the QA coordinator may discern common problems of concern to health care workers and administrators.

The Quality Assurance Nurse's Approach

- Focuses on the legal consequences of medication errors.
- Looks for trends and patterns in relation to medication in the big picture of the nursing service organization.
- Interprets trends.
- Searches to identify systems problems and seeks solutions.
- Communicates with and seeks the advice of hospital legal counsel.
- Suppresses rumors and concentrates on facts.
- Is committed to confidentiality.
- Is concerned primarily with patient safety and welfare.
- Works closely with nurse managers.
- Reacts objectively to documents and facts rather than subjectively to personal repercussions of medication errors.
- Advises hospital personnel to avoid using incident reports as a form of punishment.
- Sees medication errors as hospital crises.

RISK MANAGERS

Risk managers create and maintain programs of risk identification and control for hospitals. Their programs are guided by hospital policy and supported by hospital administration so that the effects of loss on the health care organization are contained when human, physical, and financial assets are threatened. The adverse effects of medication errors challenge the resources of the risk managers who implement the quality-control program of the institution. The success of the program is dependent on the risk manager's ability to organize and communicate the objectives of the program.

A nurse who has been a risk manager for over 11 years shared her perspectives on medication errors and her work in a community hospital. She is an experienced, thoughtful, highly professional nurse who brings her great sense of fairness and attention to detail to her work. Her story follows:

There is not a lot of research on medication errors. I think that everybody thinks that medication errors are going to happen when you are administering thousands and thousands of doses of medications. A couple of medication errors that I can think of stand out in my mind, although none had a serious outcome. There was one that involved the nursery; it took place about four years ago. The drug involved was an antibiotic.

A physician ordered a particular drug, and it was transcribed properly onto the medication cardex. However, the pharmacist misread the placement of the decimal and sent to the nursery the dosage that he thought was correct. The receiving nurse looked at it and figured that if pharmacy saw it that way, it must be right. These nurses never questioned another department. Nor did anyone take the time to call the physician. Fortunately for the baby, the physician came in by chance and the error was averted. Had the drug been administered, the baby would have received a dosage ten times that prescribed.

There was no unhappy outcome from this episode, but it pointed out to us that nursing needs to take its responsibility a lot more seriously. Nurses need to know that they have the right to question a physician or a pharmacist and to take the appropriate steps.

An error that actually happened involved Coumadin [an anticoagulant]. The dosage was written by a resident as 2.5 milligrams, but it was transcribed as 25 milligrams. (This was before the days of sending a transcribed order sheet to the pharmacy.) It was an order written on an order sheet with no carbons, and the order was transcribed onto a pharmacy request slip. Once the nurse made the error, there was no catching it until the patient showed problems. The patient bled, had a liver biopsy, hemorrhaged, and ended up with many complications. He did not die, but his hospital stay was probably about 3½ weeks longer than it should have been—all because of one dose of medication.

That was when the hospital instituted the cross-checking of dosages of heparin. It was one of the first things that we went through when we reviewed the order: who looked at the order, who read the order, who transcribed the order. If the RN does not take the time and the responsibility to go back and look at the order to make sure that what's there is supposed to be there, it can lead to a big problem.

We've had other errors when we've dealt with narcotics—for example, the narcotics counts are not right—and you have to work through the situation. When you have to report the diversion to the state board of nursing because you have nurses who are falsifying narcotics records and using narcotics themselves, it makes for a lot of unhappiness. That is an example of one situation in which I work very closely with the nursing department. As soon as there's a recognized discrepancy, we look at all of the narcotics records. The pharmacy is now very acutely aware of checking the daily sign-out sheets for what is at the bottom at the end of the count and what is recorded at the beginning.

One of the big changes that we made here was to have a tighter hold on narcotics. Narcotics diversion is very common in hospitals and easy to do. One of the nurses was very, very smart; she made sure that she always did the narcotics count. She would record at the bottom of the sheet that there were, say, 24 perfect sets of one narcotic remaining at 7:00 A.M. when the changeover in sheets takes place and write 20 at the top of the next page.

This nurse was fired, and we had to report it to the state board of nursing. She went through a nurse recovery program, the best outcome for her. Nurses who get into a rehabilitation program may be able to come back to work, although probably not in a position where they're going to have access to drugs.

We've had some positive and some negative results with the recovery program. Recently we've had a few nurses who went through the recovery program and seem to be doing just fine now. They're working in much more controlled circumstances, with fewer narcotics around and available.

We did employ a chemically dependent nurse who was a nurse anesthetist. She was fine for a year but then began to slip. She lost her job, and there is no chance for her to come back. It was much more difficult to find her pattern of diversion because she was not working on a patient unit. The anesthetists have such a free rein with the controlled drugs that they are giving and not giving, and between the pharmacy and the anesthesia department, it gets to be real loose at times. The anesthetists just come over to the pharmacy with their medication box and say they need a refill. Without doing a lot of checking, the pharmacy would refill it. Since the time of the nurse anesthetist's problem, the pharmacy has been much more accountable.

When a medication error is discovered, I conduct the preliminary investigation. Once the Coumadin error that I mentioned before was recognized, I was called. I went to the unit and interviewed the nurse in order to write down her thoughts on how she transcribed the order and what checks she went through as she transcribed it. She talked about what kinds of things were going on at the time, how she transcribed the order, what she thought of when she looked back at the order sheet to see what other dosages the person had been given, and what her understanding was of prothrombin times and the ratio and how that influences the dosage of Coumadin. What we discovered was that she had a basic lack of knowledge on the blood testing versus the dosages. If she had looked at the blood tests and understood them, she never would have given that dosage.

The family of the injured person was very understanding. They worked with us, and the error has not resulted in a lawsuit. It's past the statute of limitations, so I don't think it will. Clearly you need rapport with the family from the beginning.

We have an active patient relations department here. The department staff make themselves known to the patients and families as the patients come in, so that they are a known entity and people feel comfortable talking to them. As a risk manager, I don't usually deal with the patient and family. I guide where the incident goes and work closely with patient relations, but we don't put another player in the cards. Patient relations stays as the focus for the family to talk to.

The head of that department is an excellent facilitator. The one thing that we do together is work with the physicians to maintain rapport with the family. Lots of times when something bad happens to a patient, the physician wants to be the furthest removed from the situation. We have to make it very clear to the physician that we can't abandon the patient or the family at that point. We have to be open and upfront with them. With patient relations working through me, we've been able to keep the physician in the forefront and keep the lines of communication open.

Staff development instructors are more involved with nurses who make medication errors than I am. Sometimes the instructors have the nurse take a medication test. Each month we look at the medication error statistics that are reported, and if we find that one particular nurse is making errors regularly, we deal with it. If it is an agency nurse, we deal with the nurse through the agency. We probably don't want this person back in the institution if she's not well enough prepared. If it's an in-house nurse, the staff development instructor deals with this person. If it's a first error and the problem seems to be a lack of knowledge, the nurse can do some refresher work. If it's a new nurse who is befuddled by everything, the preceptor gets more involved.

The nurse managers keep track of any medication errors their staff make, and they have access to the incident reports. If I sense that one nurse more than another is involved in any kind of error, I call it to the attention of the nurse manager, who will do some more tracking and follow-up. The nurse manager also will look at incident reports and the performance of the rest of the staff on the unit to see what's going on with them. I try not to make the incident report a reprimand or any kind of punishment because nurses may not fill them out.

If you want good reporting of medication errors, you've got to use incident reports, but you have to use them in a discrete way. I don't see the incident report as a punishment tool. If it is used in that way, the staff nurses start viewing the risk manager as a punishment person, and they may think, "Well, if that's the way the report is going to be used, we just won't fill them out." I would rather they felt comfortable filling them out for any error, no matter how small or benign it may seem, so that at least you know what's going on in the units.

My role is not to be a punisher but to be the person who reads the reports and gets an understanding of the kinds of things that are going on, such as patient falls, med errors, or some other specific problem identified in a report. I work from there with whatever means I have. If I need to look at falls, we'll focus on falls. If I see a higher number of med errors, I work on that.

When we're getting a lot of new graduate nurses coming into the hospital in the summer months and a lot of people are being pushed through orientation, there seems to be an increase in medication errors. At that point we have staff development instructors out on the floors working with the new graduates. They work with the preceptors and try to head off any big problems. The new nurses start working in the hospitals in June, and that's when a lot of the more experienced nurses are taking vacation. So you have these new nurses working on the floors, and they are expected to function as if they have been here forever and a day. They are getting pressured beyond belief.

To make their experience a positive one, we decided to start a preceptor program. The preceptors know in advance when their new graduates are coming, and they don't plan their vacations then, so we don't have these floundering nurses upstairs. That has really decreased the number and the severity of the medication errors.

Also, the pharmacy is active in doing accountability studies to detect patterns on the floors. If they find a potential problem, they call the floor and talk to the nurse manager or the unit manager. There are many ways that you can pick up medication problems before you end up with a bad situation.

We are constantly looking at packaging and talking about packaging. It is a very big deal. At one point, the nurses were having a big problem with what sodium chloride for dilution of drugs looked like versus what the dilute heparin for heplocks looked like. The pharmacy has written to the manufacturer, and we have been able to influence a color change on the label. Up to that point, both were written in black, and you really had to make sure that you didn't pick up the wrong vial. Both are stocked, and both are stored near each other on the various units. This increases the chance for an error.

One of the things I've concluded is that there are a lot of errors that aren't recorded. But I think there are different approaches to reporting errors among hospitals. If you ask the nursing staff on a unit to fill in an incident report for every minor thing, I'd probably have a drawer full of incident reports every month, and there's no way that I could do anything effective with those. I discourage nurses from routinely reporting certain things, such as IV infiltrations with just a plain IV running. But if the IV has medications in it, obviously you want to know because there is the potential for skin damage or further damage to the area, even at some later point, depending on whether it is chemotherapy or just potassium chloride or an antibiotic or whatever.

If the nurses filled out an incident report for every IV infiltration that occurred, especially with the elderly who tend to have frail, thin veins that pop IVs out a couple of times a day, they'd do nothing but fill out incident reports. I think they have to learn to use some common sense, but also the things that need to be reported can vary from one person to another. It's better to pick up the phone and ask, "Is this something really worth reporting?" It's easy for them to do that, with somebody being here. The supervisors on the evening and night shift work closely with me, so they're pretty in tune to what we need to know.

I'm certain things go on I don't hear about, but I think the more people get used to the idea that there's a risk manager in the hospital, the more comfortable they feel developing rapport with him or her. I'm up on the floors probably at least once a day. People see me, talk to me, and feel free to ask me questions. Even if a situation doesn't come down on an official piece of paper, I get a sense of what's going on. The incident may not quite fit into the boxes on our preprinted incident report form, so the nurse may think, "Well, if it's not there, then I don't have to report it." I'd much rather they feel comfortable talking to me, and at least at that point, we would be able to initiate some type of report so that it can be followed up by the risk manager or the quality assurance person.

In relation to documenting a medication error, I recommend that the nursing staff put it in a very factual statement. If a nurse gave Dilaudid instead of Demerol, there are no big problems expected. But I'd like him to document the fact on the medication cardex—just the fact that it has been given. About nurses' notes, I can say that some people do it better than others. They write an interim note and say: "Patient given Dilaudid, 2 milligrams IM" (or IV or however it was given). They state the vital signs and make a note to watch the patient and note any reaction. End of comment. We've had a case where somebody was given a drug that he said he was allergic to. We encouraged the documentation in the patient's chart. If you don't have the documentation in the chart and you're giving care or watching the patient, you run into a big problem if the patient has the reaction that he said he might have from the drug. Now, in our case, if the patient was given a drug that he was thought to be allergic to and he did not have an allergic reaction, then he was probably not allergic to the drug. It made him a little sick to his stomach but he did not have anaphylaxis, which some antibiotics can cause.

I need that kind of thing documented. Usually as soon as I get an incident report documenting that kind of problem, I review the chart to see whether it's there. If it's not there, I ask the nurse to go back and put an interim delayed note in the charts just to record what happened and what the patient's vital signs were. There should also be a record of what the nurses observed on the rest of the shift or anything else of note. It's documented then. If someone is going to pick up on it, they're going to pick up on it from a legal standpoint. But most times it's better to have it in the chart than not have it.

When something happens, such as a medication error, I am there to make sure that this person is talking to that person. I'm one of the logical, detail-oriented people here; that is my strength in this kind of position, and it has always been the way I am. I coordinate, and I have the physicians and the families talking, whether directly through my efforts or through the patient relations department.

I certainly look at the kinds of things that are going on. I check the documentation on the medical record to make sure that it's there, that it's complete, that what needs to be in there is there and what doesn't need to be in there isn't there. When the medical record isn't complete, it will be kept in what we call our restricted pile for a certain period of time. I do this so that there is no attempt at any later date for somebody to come along and think, "I should have done this," and go back and look for something in the medical record. As soon as I know there has been a problem that has any kind of potential for a disastrous outcome, that record is kept in a secured place. Two people have the key to it, and that chart is not given out for anyone to look at without an OK from me. That does really cut down on the chances for alterations being made at a later date.

I don't usually attempt to influence the nurse manager to remove the staff nurse who made the error from the patient's case. The fact that the person who committed the error can still work with the patient lets her feel that she is still worth something as a nurse. I think it allows the patient to deal with the situation too. I can't see what's going to happen in every case. Most patients are understanding, but some families are a little less understanding. As long as the patient feels comfortable, I do not discourage the nurse from taking care of the patient. Of course, in an error of any kind, if the patient loses confidence in the nurse, you have to remove the nurse from the situation. But it's not one of my usual things to recommend. And I don't think many of the unit managers or nurse managers would unless it was apparent that there was a problem.

I report directly to the president of the hospital and have direct access to the directors and the vice president of nursing, as well as the nurse managers. I also interact with physicians a lot. I have no problems dealing with them. The more that I work with them and the more that I work through a lawsuit with them, the more comfortable they become with me. The physician I go through most often is the director of medical affairs. If I notice a lot of this type of problem or that type of problem, I tell him that I think we need to address it. I usually get a good response.

I've been here over twenty years. The physicians knew me as a nurse; now they see me in a different position. Even the younger doctors who come on staff are willing and talkative.

I participate in all orientation programs, so each time a new group of physicians come on staff, they see me. They might not see me the day they come on staff, but within the first few months of their time at the hospital, they hear about my responsibilities. They begin to realize what I can do and how I can help them and what kinds of things mean something or don't mean something.

This is a one-person department and my job works out pretty well; this is a small enough hospital. I don't know that the way I carry out my role would work at a larger hospital because there are so many places and so many units. We received an award from a hospital insurance agency because we have kept a handle on risks. The company rates the kinds of incidents in a hospital and the kinds of outcomes that result from the incidents. I work closely with insurance companies and with the hospital lawyer. People in the hospital see me as a legal person, so I get involved in doing things like guardianship and professional liability. The risk manager identifies and evaluates the exposure to liability that medication errors open up. She responds to identified risks immediately and communicates to all parties in the organization the sequence of events and controlling strategies to prevent similar events from occurring. The risk manager educates the nursing staff about the contributions of risk management to quality patient care. The manager involves the staff in the identification and correction of problems as they occur so that, in the case of medication errors, additional errors can be prevented.

Focus Points for a Risk Manager

- Determines sources of medication errors, whether systems originated or originated in lack of knowledge in hospital personnel.

- Pays close attention to narcotic count discrepancies.

- Appreciate the role of the patient relations department.

- Encourages physicians to maintain rapport with patients and families.

- Keeps open lines of communication with nurse managers, pharmacists, and physicians.

- Is attentive to facts recorded on incident reports.

- Evaluates causes of systems problems that result in medication errors.

- Encourages questions about reporting of incidents.

- Emphasizes the importance of factual documentation in patient charts and incident reports.

- Is especially cautious about confidentiality of patient charts and incident reports in events seen as high risk.

- Reports to hospital administrators and legal counsel for the hospital.

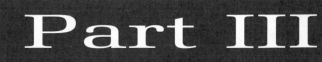

Part III

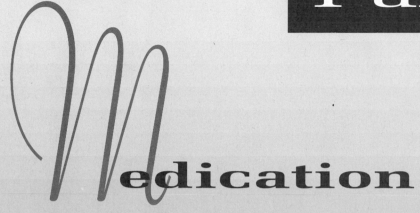

Medication Errors and Chemically Dependent Nurses

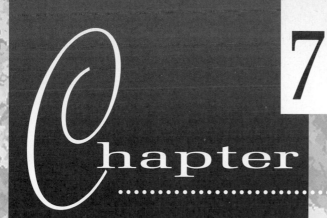

Chapter 7

Approaches to Dealing with Chemically Dependent Nurses

Nurses who divert medications ordered for patients are making medication errors. For example, a nurse may intentionally neglect to give a narcotic to a patient in pain, instead intentionally injecting sterile water or, worse, a drug that was not ordered, in lieu of the narcotic. In spite of how the error is classified, nurse managers, supervisors, and administrators bear the burden of noticing, monitoring, documenting, and acting on the problem as medications are diverted. As they gain experience with supervising chemically dependent nurses, they develop systematic approaches to confirming and confronting the problem and the nurse.

The first narrative in this section relates the experiences one nurse administrator had with chemically dependent nurses over the course of her career. Her values about patient care and managing nurse employees emerge in this story, as do the practical strategies she developed to handle the confirmation, confrontation, and aftermath phases that accompany this experience.

The second narrative comes from a seasoned director of nursing. From her experiences, she provides her perspectives on the problem of chemical dependency, diversion of controlled substances, and medication errors resulting from these situations.

THE RIGHTS OF CHEMICALLY DEPENDENT NURSES AND THE RIGHTS OF PATIENTS

When I came to that patient unit, I had a sense that there was a problem with narcotics diversion. Perhaps I was uneasy about the type of care that was being given, the attendance patterns of some of the employees, and the lax approach to dealing with narcotics and other medications. Because of this gut feeling and the fact that I had dealt with chemical dependency problems in the past, I began to observe certain nurses' practice more closely and to let the nursing management staff know that I thought that there might be a problem.

After I talked to the pharmacy technicians who deliver the narcotics to the unit, I was invited to the pharmacy—off the record—to look at the narcotics sheets that had been returned from this particular unit. I soon realized that there appeared to be a significant amount of waste of narcotics at some point or dosages signed out more frequently than what appeared to have been ordered. When I started looking at the records from approximately 5 to 6 months earlier, the two pharmacy technicians told me that there had been a problem on that unit in the past and that they had notified the pharmacists and nurse administrators of a possible substitution of tablets. Additionally, one physician had suggested to the pharmacy director that a certain nurse might have a problem because her patients were complaining of not receiving medications. To these technicians' knowledge, there had been no follow-up by nursing administration.

I was beginning to suspect the nurse they mentioned and focused more on her at first. Next, I went to the medical records department to review patient charts. I found that patients were being medicated at a different time from when the drugs were signed out and that one physician ordered three and four different types of narcotics at the same time, with no instructions as to what should be given when. It was primarily his patients' charts where I found the discrepancies. I eventually identified five nurses who appeared to have significant documentation problems.

After I spoke with the pharmacy personnel and before I confronted the nurses, I reported the situation to the clinical director, who responded, "Well, we thought there was a problem, but we looked at it and didn't see anything, so we ignored it." It became clear to me that perhaps people in the organization at the upper administrative level didn't know how to look for a narcotics problem. If it wasn't right there and jumping out—if someone didn't come forward and say, "I have a problem"—they didn't look any further because they didn't know how to.

I told the clinical director that I thought at least one nurse was chemically dependent; furthermore, I suspected a ring of people working together to divert drugs. She thought my suspicions were ridiculous but agreed to support whatever I wanted to do.

I started to collect data on the frequency of dosages being administered and noted that the dosages didn't correlate with the patients' medical records. Also, there appeared to be significant forgery and an enormous amount of narcotics that were never accounted for. When I reported this information to the clinical director, she started to buy in to my theory and assist me in reviewing the medical records. She did not delve as deeply as I did, and in a lot of records that she surveyed, she didn't see the patterns that I found. Nevertheless, she was very supportive of my efforts, and her approach to documenting the evidence of diversion was the same as mine. I think she was just a little uncomfortable to think that the problem had been an ongoing one, that people had alerted her to it in the past year, and that she didn't know how to find it or hadn't looked hard enough.

The chief nurse executive also thought that there probably was a problem but didn't know the extent of it. Her reaction was not unusual. More often than not, unless a nurse is clearly impaired in her practice and the problem is obvious to other nurses, supervisors will wait until there is something obvious—say, a dirty syringe left behind in the locker room. No one wants to take action until the problem is obvious—for example, needle marks on a nurse's arms or a nurse with glassy eyes. There are other signs as well: things that are obvious to me are sloppy documentation, changes in handwriting, and absenteeism problems before and after weekends off.

Together, the clinical director and I approached each nurse—I would never intervene alone—and said we felt that there was a significant problem with documentation. Then we reviewed all the discrepancies that we found and said that if the nurse had a problem, we could refer her to a treatment program. If the nurse denied that there was a problem, we said our only option was to terminate for cause. None of them confessed to a chemical dependency, and so all were fired.

In this sort of situation, documentation is important. The facts must clearly identify a problem, and the documentation must provide support. If a patient complains of not being medicated, for example, at some point the nurse is going to have to increase the patient's frequency of use—more frequently than what the patient requires. Sometimes you'll see meds signed out for patients who aren't there anymore. Or a nurse will sign out some days that she wasn't even at work. And sometimes you can walk into a lounge and find someone with a syringe.

This was a very difficult situation. Numerous other managers, some physicians, and other people in the organization thought that I was on a witch hunt. And since two of the three terminated nurses were LPNs, they decided that I didn't want LPNs working on the unit. Some supervisors said that I was out to get particular people. They thought these were good nurses and that there wasn't a diversion problem.

The repercussions got worse too. Within 24 hours of terminating the first two nurses, my car windows were shot out. There were calls to the hospital administration, especially by a particular physician, saying that *I* was the one who was diverting narcotics and trying to pin it on other people. The postal inspectors came to the hospital approximately 3 weeks later and requested to see one of my business cards because they had found dirty syringes in mailboxes at two different locations in the city, with business cards with my name stuck in them.

They had been forged. The handwriting of my name had been forged onto the cards, and so, we sent samples of handwriting off to the FBI in Washington for analysis. And they were going to attempt to fingerprint, but it appeared that someone had used hemostats to push the business cards into the syringes, so they probably also wore gloves. I got calls at my home, hang-up calls. Hospital administration was nervous enough about this that they offered to move me to another location. But in spite of everything, I didn't feel threatened.

I thought that a physician was also involved in the harassment—one I knew and with whom I had had a wonderful relationship. Since that time, the man hasn't looked at or spoken to me. And he's now demanding that the hospital administration put in writing that I will never be present on a unit where his patients are.

Another story that stands out in my mind occurred when I was a nurse manager on an ICU. I had only been there a month or two when it came to my attention that narcotics diversion might be taking place. I found out when I called in to the other unit that I was covering on the weekend, and someone said, "Oh, did you hear that ICU is losing narcotics again?"

In backtracking, I learned that the weekend supervisors had known about the diversion for a couple of months. They had noted that the count was off but then went ahead and cosigned and then corrected the records, and that was it. I then looked at three charts in medical records and identified who the person was with the problem. I gathered a significant amount of documentation and then pulled two tubexes from stock and had them analyzed. The drugs involved were Demerol (meperidine hydrochloride) and morphine. There was no narcotic in either of those syringes. Apparently the nurse had been replacing it with saline for a few months at least. Who knows whether any patients were injured, because you don't know what was substituted when.

The director of nursing wanted to terminate this person, but I convinced her to offer to put the nurse out on leave and get her some assistance. The nurse, however, clearly stated that she had no problem—she wasn't diverting—and she wasn't going to buy into it all. But we had copies of the documentation and suspended her, pending further investigation. We're not going to bring her back to work because we continued to uncover additional discrepancies and notified the state board of nursing. The state board never came to investigate, though, and 6 years later, I read that her license had been revoked in another state for drug and alcohol abuse.

In the first example, all the documentation that is collected in this sort of situation is sealed in a locked file, and the state board is called and told that someone has admitted to diversion or is implicated but admitting nothing. The state board then sends someone to the hospital to review the documentation with the person who collected the data. Within 2 weeks, and perhaps because I called with four names, someone from the Department of Professional Regulations came to the hospital and reviewed the documentation. However, the hospital attorney didn't want me to speak with him without a subpoena, based on all the other problems that were going on, such as the damage to my car and the dirty syringes with my business cards. He didn't want me put in the position of accusing anyone of any illegal behavior. So under subpoena, I was called down to the city to give my account and share all my documentation and my personal notes from conversations with the individuals.

When we confronted one nurse, she said, "I didn't divert drugs but this is clearly poor documentation, I'll turn my license over to you right now," and, "This is appalling, I'm not going to sit for my RN boards next week because this is a total disgrace, I should be reported to the State Board. Who do I have to call?" The following morning, she came in demanding copies of all the patient records; she stated that she had no problem, that she was accused, that she was put under pressure, and her entire story changed. She recanted her admission that the documentation was poor.

So, typically if you meet with someone the next day, you'll either find the person agreeing to get into treatment because of what the other implications are, or the person comes back with a totally different story. This most recent group of nurses seemed to have a united front. They had all gone out and gotten an attorney together.

In one case, what really began my initial investigation was a placebo order written for a patient without a physician's order. It was on the medication cardex. And the order sheet said, "May give placebo, PRN [as needed]." The LPNs took it upon themselves to clarify the order on the medication cardex, and they gave a placebo every 2 hours in place of Demerol. Then the next night they changed that, alternating with Demerol, so they were clearly writing their own orders. When I questioned them, they said, "Well, call the doctor. He'll tell you that he probably said that to us, or he'll back it up with an order." I told them that wasn't the issue. The issues were that they had written orders and weren't licensed to do so and that the patients were receiving some-·thing that clearly wasn't indicated or prescribed for them. These were medication errors. One person was suspended.

The potential effect on the patient needs to be taken into account too in relation to whether you suspend, counsel, or terminate. If I had been faced with someone who gave saline instead of Demerol, it may not have resulted in the same story because a patient is going to be in pain without the narcotic. I personally consider it to be a crime that anyone has to be in pain when there are drugs available for pain management. And a situation in which Lasix (furosemide) [a diuretic] or digoxin [a cardiac drug] is substituted for narcotics is potentially life-threatening. And I think that had those nurses been identified and confronted, I would have terminated them, but that was never explored as an alternative for solving the problem. I think you have to look at the impact that this diversion is going to have on a patient's welfare.

Another time, a nurse's work attendance problem brought the issue to my attention. I was the assistant director, and the nurse manager was going to counsel him. I asked her to pull some medication records and look at them to see if there was something else going on. I didn't know this employee, but I had heard that he was an excellent nurse—very reliable. The nurse manager thought I was a little crazy to look at medication records when he had an attendance problem, but as we worked, we realized there were some significant discrepancies.

I called the nurse and asked him not to come in to work that night. He never asked why, which is unusual. Someone calls you at 7 o'clock and tells you not to come to work, and you don't say why? The following morning, he walked in to my office and said, "I want to thank you for calling. I know why you called. Yes, I've been diverting drugs." He did say, though, that he had never diverted medications from patients who needed them for pain.

I never even had to mention it to him. Then he started crying, and he said, "I've been waiting for someone to confront me. I was begging people to confront me, and no one would do it." He had gotten caught in a cycle and couldn't get out of it. As many times as he left trails behind him, he said no one even suggested he had a problem, and he couldn't do it himself because he thought he would be terminated and couldn't support his family.

He asked to be terminated. I told him no; we would place him on a medical leave so he could get help. He agreed to go for therapy and to meet with me weekly. After he came out of this treatment program, he came back to see me, and I told him that I had continued to review his charts and had identified what I thought was some forgery. He confessed he had forged other people's names. He even identified some that I hadn't uncovered. Because he had done more than impair himself—he also put other nurses at risk—I said he could not return to this hospital. One reason was that I thought if people found out, they probably would want to lynch him. Also, I thought that he had already placed this hospital, patients, and other nurses at enough risk. I did tell him that I would give him a recommendation and say that he worked for us and that he treated patients very well.

My advice to nurses is that if they think someone has a problem and they don't feel comfortable reporting it, they should at least bring it to someone else's attention. If that person is not comfortable, then they should continue to take it through the channels. They must protect their patients. I think they need to look at what they are in nursing for. Are they not there to be a patient advocate? And someone who is impaired is putting patients at risk.

One final story comes from colleagues at the administrative level. One of the assistant directors appeared to be impaired, and everyone just accepted the fact that that was the way she was; she was out of control sometimes. After I left the organization, another nurse manager called me and said, "I really feel that this person is impaired and may even be suicidal at this point. What should I do?" I told her that she had an obligation to try to commit the person if that's what she really felt, but she needed to talk to the nurse administrator's physician. She did, but the physician said, "She's OK. I'll just give her something to calm her down." And it appeared that the physician continued to give her prescriptions. Two months later, this person committed suicide. That nurse then had to struggle with whether she had done the right thing. She knew this person was chemically dependent and didn't help her. Where do you stop? What are your obligations?

I think that we should care about nurses as much as we care about our patients. Even a nurse who is putting a patient at risk has needs to be met and needs support. I think that it is almost contradictory to tell nurses who have these sorts of problems that they are terminated because all of their benefits, and everything that probably means anything to them, is ended. Unless we support people and bring them back to continue to care for patients and contribute to the profession, we've missed something along the way.

CONFRONTING NURSES WITH THE EVIDENCE

My most recent experience with problems with chemical dependency happened just a few weeks ago. We have a drug screening policy at this hospital and as an employment condition, everyone is screened for controlled substances during the preemployment physical. All the employees of the hospital know about it. They sign an agreement and so forth. This nurse's drug screen was positive. After the specimen was verified, two of us from nursing administration sat down and talked with her about it. I guess you would have to call this a confrontation because we were really confronting the person with her dependency.

We basically pointed out the results of the drug screen to her, and she initially said she didn't know how that happened. She was completely in denial and talked only about the over-the-counter medications she was using. So we talked some more and said, "Well, could you perhaps be medicating yourself more than you think you are?" "Well, maybe a little bit," she answered. Then we just talked, and talked, and talked, and let her think, and asked her questions. Finally, after about an hour and a half, she said, "I think maybe I've been using more than I thought." Then she started getting frightened and said,

> Oh, my gosh, that person on that paper is me! That person is not somebody else, that's me! I felt OK, and I thought I was OK, but that person on that paper, those results are me! I could have hurt a patient because I didn't even know that I could have a drug level like that.

She was appalled. She was so appalled that she could have a drug level that high and not know it, and she could have harmed a patient because she wasn't aware that she was impaired in any way. That just blew her away, completely blew her away.

This was a positive interaction—one of the most positive of this sort that I've had—because she came to her own recognition of the problem. Her first worry, as soon as it hit her, was, "Oh, my God, think of what could have happened! I don't think anything ever happened, but think of what could have happened! And I can't believe that that person is really me."

Then we moved on beyond that and talked with her about what we could do for her. She actually had come to work for us on a 13-week contract. She was a traveler—a traveling nurse—so she wasn't even one of our own employees. We talked with her about the options that we had for her. What we ended up doing was talking—helping her talk with her agency. The agency helped her remain in her housing, and we helped her get assistance. She was out for only 2 weeks and came back to our state's impaired nurses program. She is now working with us, and she's doing fine.

This nurse was not a multidrug user—I think she was using codeine—and by going through the confrontation, beginning the program, and dealing with her problem—confronting it rapidly and saying, "I don't want this to be me"—the treatment was easier than it might have been otherwise.

This nurse did not particularly make me angry because she was not diverting drugs from patients. It was clearly an illness that she didn't recognize. I know that they all have illnesses when drugs are being used and diverted, but I have trouble dealing with it when I find out that nurses are diverting medications from patients for personal use or sale. They either give patients something else—maybe sterile water or unsterile substances—or do not give patients anything for their pain. Therefore, we have patients who are suffering, and they're not getting pain relief. That makes me extremely angry. Not only are these nurses impaired when they are taking care of patients, but their patients are suffering and not getting pain relief.

I have more difficulty dealing with my anger in those situations than I do in other ones. Lots of time I have confronted nurses who have done this. Actually I've had to confront somebody in that kind of situation at least six times. Basically, most of them came about because a tampering discovery led to an investigation of nurses' documentation on narcotics records. When looking at documentation in narcotics and medication administration records, you can generally put together a pattern. You might see double sign-outs on the narcotics record but only one of them documented on the medication administration record. Or you see things that don't match or extra sign-outs. Or you see particular patterns on a particular shift with a particular nurse. But you have to have a lot of documentation. You can't confront a nurse without a lot of documentation because everybody can make a documentation error. It's not something that you can see just once or twice; it has to be patterned over time. It's very painstaking, it takes a lot of time and effort, and it's not something you can do rapidly.

Once you have the documentation, you ask the nurse to explain the discrepancies. Why is it that this was administered, and yet the sign-out was 2 hours later? What happened to this dose? What happened to this waste? You have to go through each discrepancy, one by one by one. About half of the people in that situation eventually will admit it.

At least three of the people whom I've confronted—and one of them had more documentation entry problems than anybody else that I've ever confronted—never did admit to diverting drugs. I don't know what happened to them. I've also seen forgery of other people's signatures many times. That is very, very common.

All the situations I've handled involving diversion of drugs have similarities, and all have differences. There are things about all of them that stand out in my mind, especially those nurses who have a problem and finally say, "Yes, I have a problem. Yes, I did that." Watching them confront their feeling of guilt is overwhelming, absolutely overwhelming. If they're able to get past the point where they say, "Yeah, I did," and say it again and again, next they might say, "I did it because of this or because of that." Once they get past that, their sense of guilt is great since they have succumbed and should have known better as a professional. It is a very painful thing to watch—very difficult.

The other thing that stands out is that they repeatedly say that they wished they had gotten help earlier and that they know the people they worked with knew but nobody talked to them about it. Nobody confronted them; nobody said, "What is going on? What in the hell are you doing?" The others basically turned their backs and ignored them or, worse, made it easier by letting them carry the narcotics keys all the time and enabling them to become more invested in their impairment. That makes them very angry—their nurse colleagues should know better and should be able to confront them.

I've also had the opportunity to confront nurses suspected of diverting drugs when someone else was taking the lead and I was the witness. Probably the most effective confrontations I've witnessed have been guided by somebody who is gentle but firm and comfortable with silence—as much as 15 minutes of silence—and will state a fact—point out something on a paper, talk about it, or ask a very pointed question—but not accuse. This person will just state, "This is what this is. Tell me about it." During the silence, the nurse will begin to talk and have to come up with something because nobody else is talking. Some nurses, of course, never come to the point of saying, "Yeah, I did it."

I remember another situation in which documentation clearly pointed to something happening. I still don't know if the nurse was impaired or was allowing somebody else to do something with the drugs and just signing her name. But she was involved with diversion, that was clear. There was no mistaking the documentation patterns, but she couldn't, or wouldn't, explain the pages and pages and pages of documentation. She basically said, "I don't divert. It's not my problem. I'm not going to talk to you about this. And I don't have a problem." We tried every possible angle, and we couldn't get anywhere. After offering different kinds of assistance and telling her that if she did have a problem, we could help her, and if somebody else had a problem, we could help them, we terminated her employment based on her documentation practices and reported her to the state board of nursing. We received a letter from the state board that said, "Thank you very much. We have investigated this case. We agree that a section of the Nurse Practice Act has been violated; however, we do not feel that we can pursue it at this time due to our limited resources. If we feel that there are any further complaints about this person, we will follow up at that time." That answer frustrated me.

To me, there is a difference between nurses who are diverting controlled drugs and everyone else who makes a medication error. Everybody is capable of making a medication error; everybody blows it occasionally. Everybody forgets, or gives something late, or forgets to sign something out. But I think there is a difference between a medication error and the larger patterns of practice that happen over time. These I don't consider errors but willful omissions or willful alterations. These are planned actions.

It takes a long time and patience to collect the evidence on medication diversion. I think that most nurses don't want to see the signs to identify the patterns. I've seen this repeatedly in the organization where I work now. I still have difficulty convincing the majority of people in the hospital to recognize that we have a problem. And I keep telling people, and trying to educate them, and trying to demonstrate the facts. I've been trying to show them all of the things that we do to contribute to that problem—not talking about it, not talking about good practice, not confronting people, not correcting people when they practice inappropriately. The rest of us are doing all sorts of things instead of confronting the problem.

One of our biggest problems is being able to deal with our own colleagues in our profession who are ill. If we deny collectively that we have a problem, then we'll never deal with it. The biggest thing that nurses as professionals need to come to grips with is that we too are human.

Tips from Nurse Administrators on Chemically Dependent Nurses and Medication Errors

- There are three phases of dealing with a chemically dependent nurse who is diverting medications: confirmation, confrontation, and aftermath.

- Value your intuition. Notice attendance patterns, quality of nursing care, and lax handling of medications.

- Alert nursing staff, pharmacists, and administrators to your suspicions after a preliminary investigation is conducted.

- Focus on documentation: patterns of wasted narcotics and other controlled substances, mismatches between records of administration on the patient record and times of narcotic sign-outs, forged signatures, and narcotics record patterns. Be patient, data collection takes time.

- Be aware that often nurses ignore their suspicions and that only the obvious signs of chemical dependency and diversion of controlled substances net immediate action.

- Carefully review the evidence in records, and then seal it.

- If you are a staff nurse, share your concerns with your nurse manager or another trusted manager. Do not ignore the signs.

- If you are a nurse administrator, confront the nurse in the presence of a witness; use silence; present the evidence factually; offer employee assistance programs.

- Notify the state board of nurses.

- Confront your values system: a chemically dependent nurse who diverts medications causes patients to suffer and may be too ill to give safe care to patients.

- Realize that some nurses are chemically dependent; accept the fact that nurses are human.

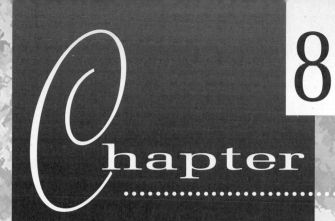

Chapter 8

Tampering with and Diverting Drugs: A Case Study

*In this chapter, a nurse administrator shares her story of an evolving sit-
uation of narcotics diversion and tampering with packaged narcotics. As
the events unfolded, she acted much like a disaster commander and
stayed on top of the situation. Her chief priority was the safety of the
patients, who were not receiving medications as prescribed.*

A nurse discovered that one box of injectable Dilaudid (hydromorphone hydrochloride) had been tampered with. When she reported
this to the nurse manager of the unit, both of them inspected other
injectable narcotics and found additional boxes bearing evidence of
tampering. The nurse manager alerted the director of nursing and the
assistant director of the pharmacy.

The seal at the bottom of the tubex boxes had been opened. When the
nurses took the tubexes out of the package, they discovered that the
boxes had been opened on the back side, at the opposite end from
which a nurse would normally open the box and pull the syringes out.
Nurses ordinarily would not be inclined to turn over the package to
look at the back. The package has clear, tough cellophane on it that is
difficult to pierce. A sharp instrument had been used to penetrate the
bottom of the box so that the narcotics could be removed and another
substance inserted after tampering. The tampering was clever; the
boxes looked as if they had been glued back together again.

When the nurse manager, pharmacist, and director of nursing examined the plungers on the tubex syringes, they noticed that they were
positioned at different levels and concluded that the syringes had been
filled up again, since there was liquid in them. They noticed another
indicator of tampering when the sheaths on the needles were removed:
the nurse manager pulled the sheaths off easily and heard no sound of
suction.

Two of the boxes that were tampered with were sent to the hospital
laboratory for analysis. Over the next week, before the results of the
analysis were returned, the director of nursing and nurse manager
ordered an audit of the narcotics sheets in search of discrepancies. As
they glanced through the sheets, they saw that someone was signing
out a large amount of narcotics. This was not very surprising, since the
unit served surgical patients exclusively.

A pharmacy technician who normally conducted routine inspections
of the unit's handling of narcotics conducted an audit. He was
instructed to inspect everything in the narcotics drawer and found ten
additional boxes of narcotics that had been tampered with using the

same method. The director of the pharmacy and the nurse manager agreed that the tampered boxes of narcotics should be replaced immediately and told the staff, by way of explanation, that there was a recall of the medications by the manufacturer.

At this point, the directors of the security and legal departments were notified, and they met with the director of nursing, one administrator from the pharmacy, and the nurse manager of the unit to come up with strategies to address the situation. They also decided to check the narcotics drawer on the other side of the unit and found four more boxes that showed evidence of tampering.

At this point, the pharmacy technician who knew about the tampering decided to check the narcotics sign-out sheets against pharmacy dispensing records. He found that three boxes of narcotics had been dispensed from the pharmacy but were not recorded on the unit's daily narcotics sheet.

It was common practice for nurses to go to the pharmacy for additional narcotics when demand on the unit was high. One of the nurses would take the daily narcotics sheet to the pharmacy and request the narcotics. The pharmacist would then record the additional medications dispensed on the top of the sheet and add them to the unit's tally, sign his name, and ask the nurse to sign to indicate receipt of the additional drugs. But in this case, there was no record of the additional narcotics being dispensed to the unit, in conflict with the pharmacy's record of the transaction.

The nurses speculated that a dummy sheet had been taken to the pharmacy. Each unit had blank forms on hand for the times additional narcotics were needed. The person who diverted the narcotics filled in the sheet so that it looked authentic to the pharmacist, and the narcotics never made it to the unit.

It was not long before the nurses discovered that four more boxes bore evidence of tampering. These had been returned to the pharmacy from another unit. It now appeared that the extent of the tampering was widespread.

In their investigation, the nurse manager and the director of nursing began to notice discrepancies in one particular nurse's documentation, but they carefully reviewed the performance of all nurses assigned to the unit and reflected on any recent changes in behavior. They discussed nurses who had family and money problems and wondered if any of the staff had a chemical dependency.

Next, the director and manager obtained a list of names of the nursing staff who had worked when the drugs were dispensed by the pharmacist to the unit and asked the pharmacist to describe the individual who had signed out the additional narcotics. The description he provided roughly matched the nurse whom the director and manager suspected of diverting the narcotics.

After another audit of the narcotics sheets, the nurse manager and director again pinpointed the same suspected nurse. Further, the manner in which this nurse had documented narcotics administration suggested chemical dependency. For example, one narcotics sheet revealed that a single patient was supposed to have received two doses of an intramuscular narcotic within 45 minutes and, later in the shift, another two doses, purportedly given to that patient 1 hour apart. Additionally, the patient was ordered less narcotic than the nurse had signed out, and none of the narcotics doses were recorded as wasted. When other patient charts were audited, the same pattern was evident. That same nurse also had signed out a narcotic for doses for which there were no orders, and nothing in the nurse's note on the record pointed to the patient's having extraordinary pain or suffering. It was also clear that several narcotics were involved or diverted.

Although the nurse suspect appeared to be diverting an oral medication as well, the administrators focused on the injectable medications because of the evidence of tampering. As the situation evolved, more boxes of tampered narcotics were discovered.

The nurse manager and the director of nursing convinced the legal department to inform a charge nurse who worked on the same shift as the suspected nurse. The charge nurse was in a better position to check the narcotics drawer more often than the nurse manager, who had been checking it once daily to detect additional tampering. Over the course of the week and weekend, six additional tampered boxes were found. The nurse manager and the director of nursing noticed that a few of the same nurses were working every time the administrators discovered tampering.

The chief nurse executive (CNE) was aware of these events as well. The director of nursing had shared her concerns with the CNE about whether the patients on the unit were being provided adequate patient care. It was evident to all of the informed nurses that medications were being withheld from patients, and because the laboratory analysis on the syringes originally discovered was not yet completed, they worried about whether patients were receiving narcotics as prescribed. The CNE shared her fear with the director about whether the suspected nurse was injecting herself with needles from tampered syringes and later reusing the same needle to inject the patient. All of the informed nurses had serious concerns about the patients' pain relief, and they could foresee a situation in which a patient complained about not getting relief, the physician prescribing the medication, and the patient receiving excessive narcotic.

The CNE and the director were having difficulty convincing the legal and security directors that safe patient care was a serious concern. Both nurses recognized that although these administrators were concerned with patient safety and pain relief, they also needed to focus on fact finding and the chain of evidence. The legal counselor and director of security, however, thought that they did not have all of the facts yet and considered it premature to take any action. After several frustrating days, the director of nursing and the CNE were able to convince counsel and the security chief that the suspected nurse had to be confronted. The scope of the diversion may have been wide, and it could have been taking place for an extended time.

Just as the decision to confront the suspected nurse was made, she called in sick and did not come to work. While she was out, the narcotics drawers were checked every 8 hours for evidence of tampering and diversion. That no additional tampering was discovered incriminated the suspected nurse even more. Further, her behavior at this time also fueled suspicions. She spoke hysterically to the charge nurse on the telephone and reported being under excessive stress. The charge nurse feared that the suspect was suicidal.

While this nurse was out, it appeared that another member of the nursing staff might be involved. It was evident that someone was bringing information to the suspected nurse when she was absent from work, and the charge nurse thought that the second nurse knew about her friend and co-worker's problem.

The nurse manager finally convinced the suspected nurse to seek assistance for her problems from the hospital's employee assistance program. She made an appointment, and the nurse manager, the director of nursing, and legal counsel were scheduled to be present when she arrived, to confront the nurse. But this plan fell through when the group decided to hold off confronting the nurse. Nursing and the legal department went back and forth indecisively the following week. The nurse was present in the hospital a few times to attend sessions provided by the employee assistance program, but she did not work on the unit, and no confrontation took place.

Finally, the legal department and the director of nursing agreed the time to confront had arrived, and when the suspected nurse next came to the hospital to attend another meeting with an employee assistance counselor, the director of nursing and the nurse manager brought her to the nurse administrator's office and asked her to explain the discrepancies in narcotics documentation.

The nurse began by pointing out that the medications had been ordered, that the resident physicians had forgotten to write the orders, that they had given the nurse verbal orders, and that the patients on the unit had received many narcotics. Then the director of nursing asked why the nurse had consistently signed out narcotic analgesics at the beginning of the shift. The suspected nurse explained that she always medicated patients at the beginning of the shift: "Well, I always come on, and everybody gets pain medication, so I always thought, give them their pain medication."

The director of nursing was steadfast in her repeated confrontation of the nurse with the facts. Several times she insisted that the nurse explain the discrepancies in documentation and encouraged the nurse to talk to her about her personal situation. She also pointed out that the documentation audit indicated a chemically dependent person and assured the nurse that she would help her get into a treatment program. She also told the nurse that she would be suspended pending the investigation and most likely would be terminated at the hospital because of poor nursing practice.

The nurse finally admitted that she had a problem and that she was dealing with a lot of stress in her life. She admitted that she had obtained the narcotics by signing out more than patients were ordered and used the remaining amount; or she gave patients half of the ordered dosage. However, she assured the director of nursing that she had been diverting narcotics for only a few weeks. She would not admit to tampering with the injectable narcotics and did not agree that she had obtained narcotics directly from the pharmacy. There was some doubt about the latter diversion; the pharmacist could not positively identify the nurse when he looked at the pictures of the nurses who had worked that day.

The nurse manager and director of nursing agreed that they were not sure that the problems on the unit were settled. Although the nurse was being counseled by the employee assistance program and was given a medical leave, she would be allowed to return to work after several weeks following participation in the state's chemically dependent nurses' program. The director of nursing reported the nurse to the state board of nursing and expected her to attend the chemically dependent nurses' program. The nurse was obligated to call the program.

Finally, when the legal department representatives interviewed the nurse, she was surprised to be confronted with the tampering allegations. The nurse manager and director of nursing were unsettled about this. Too many narcotics had been diverted. Finally, there was additional proof of problems; both the hospital laboratory and the outside laboratory confirmed that there was evidence of tampering.

The story did not end here, since the director of nursing was fully aware that she continued to have a problem on her hands, as did the hospital. Additional documentation discrepancies appeared on different units. The legal department was pursuing the problem. The pharmacy and nursing departments, in response to this experience, joined forces to work on systems designed to limit diversion of narcotics. Identification badges would be required, and dispensing procedures would be revamped. Nursing and pharmacy were also looking into alternative manufacturers that supplied medications in more tamper-proof packaging. The director of nursing planned to alert all nurse managers to this experience so that they would watch their stores of narcotics more carefully.

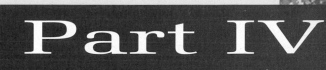

Part IV

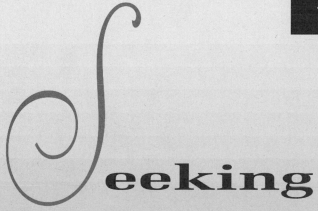

Seeking Solutions

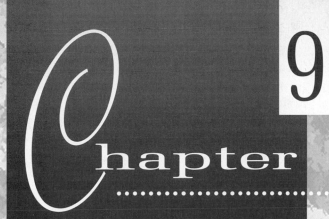

Chapter 9

Reducing the Risks Associated with Medication Errors

Many hospitals have developed programs designed to prevent medication errors from happening or to react to mistakes that have been made. This chapter contains advice that is guided by a teaching plan created to reduce the incidence of medication errors (Appendix B) and to minimize the effects of medication errors after they occur. Appendix C includes an instructional booklet designed to assist nurses to learn to manage the risks associated with medication errors.

DEFINING MEDICATION ERRORS

A medication error is defined as a mistake made at work in administering drugs ordered by physicians and dispensed by pharmacists. The patient either receives a medication incorrectly or fails to receive it. Medication errors are thus unintentional mistakes that involve the prescription, transcription, dispensing, or administration of drugs and IV solutions. Nurses cite medication errors as follows: wrong patient, wrong medication, wrong dose, wrong time, wrong route of administration, or wrong rate of administration.

There are two types of errors. A medication error of omission occurs when a nurse unintentionally fails to give a prescribed drug. An error of commission is made when a nurse gives a patient a drug that was not prescribed or an excessive dose of a prescribed medication.

Different degrees of harm can occur to a patient when errors of omission or commission are made. Death is the worst harm. Next on the scale is the presence of symptoms, a change in the patient's condition, or morbidity. Sometimes there are no noticeable results following a medication error, and occasionally the patient's condition actually improves.

Indexes of severity have been developed at some hospitals to gauge the harm incurred by medication errors. In certain hospitals, nurses get points or a score when they make these mistakes, and the numerical rating becomes part of their performance record. Nurses who accumulate evidence of a pattern of medication errors may be fired because of obvious concerns for patient safety.

Whether a medication error is labeled as such may involve a subjective judgment on the part of the nurse. The definition of a medication error is confounded by many gray areas, such as the one nurses describe as the "magic hour." In this case, an error may technically have occurred, yet the nurse decides not to label it as one. For example, an iron supplement is ordered at 10 A.M., 2 P.M., and 6 P.M. A patient goes to an appointment in the physical therapy department, and the nurse gives the medication at 8 A.M., not 10 A.M. It is iron, so the nurse thinks that it makes sense to give it with breakfast. But the nurse does not take the time to ask the physician to write the order that way or to write the time that the medication was actually given in the medication admin-istration record. This kind of situation, in which there is a deviation from the prescription, is common and does not constitute an error in the eyes of most nurses.

A nurse who is involved in this sort of situation has not violated any-thing in terms of patient safety; in fact, the nurse added good judgment to a situation that the physician was unaware of or had not thought through carefully. The nurse then has to decide whether to fill out an incident report. The answer may be no; the nurse determines that the situation does not result in severe harm, so the error is not a problem.

Many nurses also use the criterion of harm in deciding whether an error has been made. They might give the wrong drug but decide it is not a medication that could cause the patient harm. For example, for-getting to give digoxin is considered a serious problem; forgetting to give Tagamet (cimetidine) is not. The patient might suffer from not get-ting the Tagamet, but a nurse might not consider the omission to be serious.

On the other hand, to bend the rules day after day is not sensible. Good judgment requires speaking with the physician and getting the order and the situation changed. Moreover, it is difficult to explain the rules to nursing students and graduate nurses when the extenuating circumstances of nursing practice encourage seasoned nurses to bend them.

Hospitals have policy and procedure manuals that detail the rules gov-erning medication administration, and most nurses certainly know what these manuals say. But they also point out that some of these policies are unrealistic:

> It often goes like this. A policy and procedure manual may say that a nurse can give a medication 30 minutes before or 30 minutes after the time that it is ordered. While this hour is aimed at by most nurses, the reality of the clinical situation dictates that this is often not possible. For example, a nurse is responsible for ten patients, five of whom are to receive insulin at 8 A.M. Change-of-shift report starts at 7:30 A.M. and ends about 8:15 A.M. How realistic is it to think that the nurse could

administer the five insulin injections in 15 minutes? Perhaps insulin should be scheduled for 8:30 A.M., since breakfast trays begin arriving at that time.

It may be difficult for nurses to adhere to the time limits set forth in a medication administration procedure because different patient units have different time constraints and patient care issues. It may be harder to meet the time restrictions set forth in the procedure than many nurses realize. Nevertheless, nurses need to be aware that policies and procedures are standards of practice. A lawyer involved in a malpractice suit would scrutinize the policy and procedure of a hospital and point out the discrepancies between the standard and the medication error incident if a patient received insulin too late and patient harm resulted.

THE STANDARD OF CARE

As we have seen throughout this book, most nurses equate good nursing practice with error-free practice. When they make a medication error, they often believe they are not doing a good job and are aware on many levels that the ethical principle of doing no harm has been violated. For example, the Nightingale pledge, written in 1893, contains an explicit warning to avoid medication errors. "I will abstain from whatever is deleterious and mischievous, and will not take or knowingly administer any harmful drug."

Nurses' concern with avoiding harm is linked with their explicit strategies to maintain patient safety. It is clear that patient safety is of great concern to them, as is the interest of nurses in providing quality care. Nevertheless, it may be impossible for nurses to avoid making medication errors, even though this is the standard that has been set.

ACKNOWLEDGING MEDICATION ERRORS

The belief that even one error is unacceptable may influence how accountable some nurses are when they make medication errors. Because punishment, not discipline, may be meted out to nurses who make medication errors, many nurses admit that they neglect to report all but the most serious errors and will not "rat" on one another. In contrast, others write incident reports frequently.

When nurses fill out incident reports, they begin to pay for their mistakes in the presence of their fellow nurses and other health care workers. In some hospitals, the reports, posted at the nurses' station, detail the events surrounding the error.

All methods of reporting medication errors serve to purge the "sin." The nurse and all other involved persons share the responsibility.

In either admitting responsibility for an error or not acknowledging the occurrence of an error, nurses control their practice. By exerting this control, they have the power to determine what is an error and when an error exists. Of course, regardless of whether the nurse admits the error, it has taken place. Admitting that a mistake happened, that something has gone wrong, is an acknowledgment of a mistake and a warning to the nurse to try to improve care.

RESPONDING TO MEDICATION ERRORS

American nurses have been indoctrinated to believe there is little or no tolerance for medication mistakes. The socialization of nurses into their role is very powerful, so much so in the case of medication errors that some nurses, having made them, carry their burdens for many years. They continue to feel very guilty and bad about themselves, even if the mistake results in minor consequences for the patient.

A nurse who has made a medication error may question whether nursing is the right profession. Nurses may develop personal rituals and routines to prevent future errors. For example, they carry notes to remind themselves about a medication, tape checklists on the medication cart, or use index cards in the medication cardex to tickle their memories. Others avoid unwrapping packaged oral medications until they carry them to the patient; then they check the drugs one at a time by reading the package in which the medication is wrapped, as they give the patient the drug. Some nurses pull the medication cardex a bit out of its place when something is unusual about a patient's medications. It helps them to notice that patient's medication record.

LIABILITY

Administrators are clear that policies and procedures serve as guidelines for employees of hospitals. When a mistake occurs, the institution can be liable, the nurse can be liable, the nurse manager can be liable, and the nurse administrator can be liable because all participate in the chain of responsibility and accountability.

Hospital policy and procedure manuals give directions to nurses,

physicians, and pharmacists on how and to whom to report medication errors. All hospitals use incident reports and publish policies
directing nurses and physicians about their responsibility.

In addition to policies and procedures, there is another part of the
paper trail addressing medication errors in hospitals. At times, nurse
administrators and managers write memos that remind staff to follow
policy and procedure or that clarify or expand policy and procedure.

When reporting a medication error, nurses have to be cautious about
what they write about the mistake in the hospital records. Facts should
be reported objectively because the documents will provide evidence
in future litigation. The hospital needs to protect the patient, and it
also needs evidence that action was taken in case of lawsuits.
Generally, many problems arise if nurses and others try to cover up
these mistakes, or delay in taking action to correct them, or take action
but forget to document the interventions. Failing to document what
actions were taken after a medication error is discovered results in
more severe judgments against nurses and other health care providers
in courts of law.

Most medication incidents that are involved in lawsuits are labeled
negligence, although a few may be classified as felonies. For example,
a nurse may intentionally give patients Pavulon (pancueonium bromide), a neuromuscular blocker that paralyzes skeletal muscle, and
then play hero by resuscitating them. There have been deaths reported
because of intentional acts involving medications. The nurses who
intentionally perform such acts may be arrested and tried in courts of
law.

DEALING WITH NURSES WHO MAKE ERRORS

Nurse administrators and managers are responsible for counseling and
educating employees who make medication errors. Usually they want
to give second chances or even third chances to those who make these
errors. Sometimes, though, they must terminate employees. There are
policies governing employee counseling, but there may not be consistent approaches to handling nurses who make several medication
errors.

The nurse manager, the director of nursing, and the director of nursing
responsible for staff education are the most concerned—and the most
accountable—administrators. Along with staff nurses, they see a med-

ication error incident through from beginning to end. In most hospitals, they oversee the formal education provided for nurses, including that concerned with medications, generally provided during a nurse's orientation, just after coming to the hospital. Also, administrators supervise graduate nurses when administering medications.

In addition to the efforts of staff development instructors, there may be additional pharmacology content presented during classes held by nurses working in different clinical areas. Some hospitals have developed self-paced learning packages to be used by nurses after they make medication errors. In some agencies, this serves as disciplinary action. However, nurses can use the review as reparation or punishment for making the error.

Hospital and nursing administrators recognize that their foremost responsibility is to protect the safety of patients. Each department's quality assurance coordinator and the nurse managers scrutinize reported medication errors for each nursing unit. Risk managers examine the incidence of medication errors hospital wide. Some risk managers are lawyers whose prime consideration is assessment of hospital liability.

Nurse managers deal directly with the nursing staff involved in the medication error. Some managers make judgments based on the attitude of the nurse toward the medication error. They will not tolerate a nurse's indifference to an error. They also view very negatively a nurse who repeatedly makes errors that do not amount to clinically noticeable changes in the patient and says, "Oh, well this is nothing." They expect that individuals will show their concern about the error. Although nurses who make medication errors may not admit that they wish to be punished, they tend to feel better if they have to do something to atone for their mistake.

Many nurses depend on others, particularly pharmacists and physicians, to pick up errors. But nurses have to acknowledge their own responsibility for their own actions (although certainly physicians and pharmacists share the responsibility for safe medication administration with nurses).

CONSEQUENCES OF MEDICATION ERRORS

For patients who are hurt, the repercussions—increased suffering, a prolonged hospital stay, and even death—can be devastating. And if a patient dies as a result of a medication error, many others suffer throughout their lives. Patients suffer social and economic harms as well. A patient who remains in the hospital longer because of a medication error is separated from family for longer. Moreover, the family may lose income if a breadwinner does not come home when expected.

A nurse who makes an error may find that colleagues no longer trust her. This nurse may be plagued with self-doubt and even become so depressed that suicide is considered.

Distrust increases among all fellow nurses if one of their co-workers continues to make medication errors. Moreover, a nursing unit may get a bad reputation as the news of high error rates spreads rapidly through the hospital.

There are monetary costs following certain medication errors: for additional medications, nursing care hours, equipment, and supplies. Furthermore, legal costs incurred by suits tax the hospital and the plaintiff. The reputation of the hospital may suffer if it is seen by the public as an unsafe place.

CONTAINING THE RISK

Reporting Medication Errors

So that nurses, physicians, and pharmacists can identify problems, medication errors must be reported. Some nurses are very conscientious and report every error they make or discover; others report an error only when they anticipate harm resulting from the mistake. They share the error verbally with other nurses individually, during change-of-shift report, and during staff meetings.

An incident report, a written report of a medication error, ideally is written factually by the nurse discovering the error. (Other types of written reports are nurses' notes, which contain evidence of medication errors, and the medication administration record, which includes documentation that a medication was not given or that another one was.)

There are some helpful guidelines in the literature about how to record facts pertinent to medication errors. Nurses should be careful to report facts and not to record names of involved hospital personnel; attributing blame in an incident report is inappropriate. Nurses should be certain to address the problem and specify the nursing interventions, to document that the patient was monitored and cared for. It should be evident that the patient's vital signs were measured and recorded. Failing to document the fact that a nurse acted after an error and in response to it suggests that the nursing staff did not acknowledge that the medication error took place. If it appears that the error was ignored, as if it never happened, nurses and others appear negligent about their care of the patient.

It is through verbal and written reports of medication errors that quality assurance coordinators and risk managers become aware of hospital problems and threats to patient safety. The flow sheets that have been created to keep the number of errors by unit before the eyes of nurse managers, clinical directors, risk managers, and quality assurance personnel help all administrative personnel to be informed.

The Risk Management Department

The purpose of risk management departments is to survey risks to the hospital and try to contain them. Risk managers scrutinize the evidence, track the problems, and try to advise nurse managers who are in close contact with nurses who make medication errors about what to do.

Risk managers also keep their eyes on hospital-wide error and other incident rates. They note other medication-related incidents, such as medication discrepancies that do not involve patients—for example, the unexplained disappearance of some controlled drugs. They understand the legal implications of these risks or errors.

The size of the risk management department depends on the size of the institution. There might be a single risk manager in a small hospital and a team of people in a large hospital. Many risk management departments report directly to the chief executive officer of the hospital, underscoring the seriousness of their charge.

Determining What Can Be Done

Hospital administrators subscribe to a zero tolerance rule—medication errors should never occur—out of fear of harming patients and concern for the liability issues that follow. But the zero tolerance rule is violated often, since it is a human tendency to make mistakes. Moreover, some of these are random errors, and it may be impossible to eliminate these entirely. Systems errors, however, are amenable to correction. For example, if nurses notice that errors result during the transcription phase of medication administration, they can work to eliminate the problems in the system. Another example of a systems problem that often results in medication errors is that different intravenous medications have labels that are similar in appearance. Manufacturers need to standardize labels on the same drugs. Some pharmacists are working on this systems problem by developing common approaches to printing labels.

WHEN A MISTAKE HAPPENS

It is good advice to notify the charge nurse and the nurse manager about a medication error as soon as possible. The physician should be called immediately; at times the pharmacy should be notified so that pharmacists are alerted to the problem; and other departments, such as risk management, should be also notified. It may not be a good idea to inform other nurses about the error. The advice that some nurses give may be misguided.

Medication errors should be documented in various records: the incident report, nurses' notes, and the medication administration record. Just the facts should be recorded; no blame should be attributed, and the names of involved personnel should not be mentioned. The nurse should document the facts of the error in the incident report as soon as possible and keep a running note of the patient's progress.

It may not be a good idea to assign the nurse who made the medication error to the involved patient, especially if the patient suffers harm as a result. Moreover, some nurses may be so troubled by the error that they lose their clinical objectivity. In addition, in the case of the serious medication error, it may be helpful to assign a "disaster commander" who keeps careful watch on the patient's progress and keeps the risk managers and administrators informed.

LIMITING FUTURE ERRORS: STRATEGIC ADVICE

Nurse-Devised Protections

Among the various protections against making medication errors that nurses have devised is the time-honored "three-time check" to prevent them from making medication errors. Over the years, nurses have incorporated variations into the check. They read the medication cardex, select the medication from the drawer in the medication cart, read the medication label as they place it in a medicine cup, and read it again at the patient's bedside as they prepare to give it to the patient. Then, they concentrate on the "five rights" as a check: the right medication in the right dose is given to the right patient at the right time by the right route of administration.

Additional protection is provided as nurses follow the policies and procedures governing medication administration. Nurses do not always read these manuals, since they are not stimulating reading. But the advice set out in these books may guard nurses from making errors.

Many nurses develop their own rituals as protection. For example, if they have made an error associated with a drug added to an IV, they tend to be very careful and run through a routine before giving that drug again by that route. Another routine is to start to give medications from the lowest-numbered room that they are responsible for and gradually working up to the highest-numbered room.

In different hospitals, the morning insulins are given by the night shift nurses before they leave the unit; in fact, some give all of the 8 A.M. medications except the insulins, and the day shift nurses give the insulins. These variations relate to the times that the breakfast trays are served and other factors. Nurses adapt to different situations and factors so that the care they give patients is as safe as possible.

Verbal Orders

Verbal orders given by a physician to a nurse that include a medication prescription can result in medication errors. Nurse administrators are especially sensitive to the problems associated with verbal orders involving medications. For example, a physician might give a verbal order over the telephone or in person and later deny giving the order at all. In this situation, it is especially important for the nurse to follow policy and procedure. One form of self-protection is to get another nurse to witness the order or to listen to the order at the same time. Another way is to repeat the order twice and ask the physician to confirm its correctness. Physicians are expected to sign the order as soon as they come to the hospital—within 24 hours of the dated, timed order.

Nurses generally do not like to take verbal orders except in an emergency situation. However, they know that extenuating circumstances arise; also, a resident physician often covers many patients at night or an attending physician could be scrubbed for surgery.

Some nurse administrators believe that when a medication error happens, the nurse did not follow policies and procedures on medication administration. Others disagree, asserting that errors happen in spite of the fact that the nurse thought that she was following procedure.

Understanding Medications

Keeping up with new pharmaceuticals can be daunting. Nurses rely on up-to-date drug books that are kept on each unit, including the *Physicians' Desk Reference*. Often when a new drug comes to the unit, the nurses look it up together and pass the information on. The hospital formulary and pharmacists are helpful in this regard. Drug incompatibility charts are also helpful but soon become outdated. Software packages are being developed to help nurses, physicians, and pharmacists check on drug incompatibilities.

Patients can be allergic to medications and have cross-sensitization to related medications. One example is a penicillin allergy that cross-sensitizes with keflex (cephalexin monohydrate). If a patient has not had a particular medication before, the nurse should be alert for an allergic reaction.

Drug interactions are also difficult to be alert to. Often nurses are aware of the interactions between drugs that they commonly administer on a specific nursing unit; it is more difficult to remain knowledgeable about potential drug interactions when new medications are ordered.

Nurses should check with a hospital pharmacist before crushing medications and mixing them with food for patients who have difficulty swallowing or mixing them with water and giving them through a nasogastric or other tube. Frequently a pharmacist may be able to provide the same medication in a suspension. This sort of modification should be cleared with the physician, since it alters the original intent of the medication order. Nurses should not automatically assume that if a medication is ordered in tablet form for oral administration, it can be crushed and given via a tube.

Nurses seldom have their knowledge and skills sharpened formally on new medications and medication administration. Drug calculations are reviewed during unit-specific in-service education programs. No one except staff development instructors comes up to nurses and says, "Do you still know how to calculate your IV medications?"

It may be helpful to develop mandatory medication reviews and calculation practice or to obtain those that other nurses have developed. Modules could be written on a unit-specific basis to cover common and new medications in order to keep nurses up-to-date.

Between these updates, nurses can seek medication knowledge from clinical specialists, physicians, pharmacists, each other, the hospital formulary, and drug books. Sometimes drug companies bring in-service programs to patient units.

Nurses acknowledge that patients may be the first to alert them to a problem. Wise nurses do not push their personal opinion on the patient or insist that they are right and the patient is wrong. There have been instances in which nurses have insisted and have ended up making a medication error. One rule that serves some nurses in this situation is "When in doubt, don't." A patient's uncertainty should plant uncertainty in the mind of the nurse.

Nurses can use their clinical judgment to determine whether giving a medication, even one ordered by a physician, could be considered an error. For example, a patient's condition gradually deteriorates; his kidneys are failing, and he is unable to excrete a medication that he has been receiving for some time. As his nurse becomes aware of this problem, she decides to stop administering the medication and rapidly notifies the physician. In another situation, a nurse may notice some symptoms and begin to suspect an adverse drug reaction. Seasoned nurses are more secure than neophytes in their handling of these situations and, because of their clinical expertise, are in a better position to avoid such medication errors.

Another opportunity for medication errors is present during the transcription from the physician's order sheet to the medication administration record and pharmacy slips. First, the physician writes the medication order. Then the medical clerk or the nurse transcribes the order and signs it off. The unit clerk's transcription is checked by the registered nurse. The next checkpoint takes place when the night nurse performs the 24-hour check. In addition, the nurse who prepared the medication for administration has the opportunity to check the transcription. Because of the flurry of activity of a busy patient unit, mistakes can be overlooked in spite of these checks.

Another strategy that nurses use to prevent medication errors is to read labels on drug packages carefully. Nurses find themselves picking up lidocaine instead of potassium because the labels are similar. Similar drug names cause medication errors too. And many times nurses do not realize that medications come in different strengths.

Potassium is one medication that deserves special notice, especially when ordered by the IV route. Many medication errors involve potassium chloride (KCl). If KCl is given directly IV, undiluted, cardiac arrest and death can result. Heparin and KCl labels have been very similar in the past, and this labeling has been associated with serious medication errors. Medications that are ordered frequently, such as every 2 hours, are also implicated in medication errors.

Nurses should question a sudden and excessive increase in medication dosage or a sudden change to more frequent times of medication administration. These changes signal a potential problem and are worth checking. Also, if nurses find themselves drawing up medication from many vials of injectable medication or pouring out many tablets, this is also a signal that a mistake could be taking place. Other warnings that a medication error has been made are the accumulation of medications in a patient's drawer in the medication cart and the accumulation of bags in the medication refrigerator of refrigerated IVs with medications added.

General Cautions

It has been suggested that a nurse's medication error rate increases on the first or second day back after being off work. In addition, nurses need to be cautious about medications that are ordered during change-of-shift report. Keeping short the response time (the time interval between the physician's medication order and the time that the patient receives it) may help to avoid a medication error. Any medication that is in a defective package or has a blurred or marred label should be returned to the pharmacy. And it is always wise to question orders that are unclear or illegible or that have part of the notation missing.

Guidelines for Preventing Medication Errors and Reducing Risks Associated with Medication Errors

- Accept personal responsibility for your knowledge of medications (actions, dosage, side effects, and so on) and your skill in medication administration.

- Keep incident reports and other documents concerning medication errors in confidence. Do not display them in public places.

- Notify physicians when orders need to be changed if patient circumstances warrant changes. Do not bend the rules.

- Follow hospital procedures covering medication administration. Also follow routines, rules, and personal rituals.

- Focus on the details of medication administration; resist paying attention to distractions.

- Recognize that medication administration procedures serve as practice standards.

- Report medication errors; do not cover them up.

- Document actions taken following a medication error; remember that documentation serves as evidence.

- Encourage physicians to give written orders rather than verbal orders. Take verbal orders only in emergencies.

- Pay close attention to patients' allergies.

- When in doubt, call the physician or pharmacist, and listen to the patient.

- Attend in-service education programs on medication administration in order to update knowledge of new pharmaceuticals. Take a dosage calculation test yearly.

- React seriously to medication errors that you and other nurses make. Do not be indifferent. Appreciate the fact that you are human and humans make mistakes.

- Be consistent and evenhanded in applying the procedures for employee counseling when reviewing staff nurses' medication errors.

- Work together with other departments to eliminate systems-related medication errors.

- Take complaints about medication packaging problems that lead to medication errors to manufacturers.

- Be especially careful about medications ordered during change-of-shift report.

- Move rapidly to administer a medication following the physician's order.

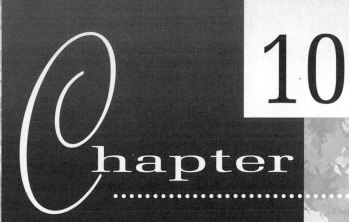

Chapter 10

A Model of Nurse-Made Medication Errors

Few individuals or institutions have formally defined medication errors, but many nurses and pharmacists have collected data on the drugs involved in the error, the units on which the events took place, and other indicators that fed into the error. Nurse managers and staff nurses pay attention to medication error rates reported by nurses responsible for quality assurance. Nevertheless, tracking systems need to be better used than they are, and they need to be aimed at monitoring trends in these errors. Prospective risk-reduction strategies need to be identified and aimed at preventing errors and reducing the risks following errors. Some think that hospitals and other health care institutions should pool their data on medication errors so that common problems can be fully described and then addressed by correcting systems problems that lead to errors.

The purpose of the model in Figure 10-1 is to show the placement of medication errors in the larger context of medication incidents and to differentiate these errors from medication discrepancies. It serves as a classification scheme to enable nurses to sort types of medication incidents. The model was constructed initially to depict medication errors as described by nurses during a study of nursing rituals and after a review of the nursing, pharmacy, and medical literature related to drug errors, additional studies on medication errors, and critiques by nurses and other health care providers. The model compares medication errors, which are patient related, to medication discrepancies, which are nonpatient-related (for example, narcotics stolen from the pharmacy).

Medication errors are either detected or undetected by the nurse making them. Of those medication errors that are detected, some are reported, and others are not. There are two major subcategories of medication errors: errors of commission, when unprescribed medication is inadvertently given to the patient or when a prescribed medication is given in the wrong dose, wrong route, and so on; and errors of omission, when prescribed medication is inadvertently not given to the patient.

Figure 10-1
A Model to Depict Medication Errors

MEDICATION INCIDENTS

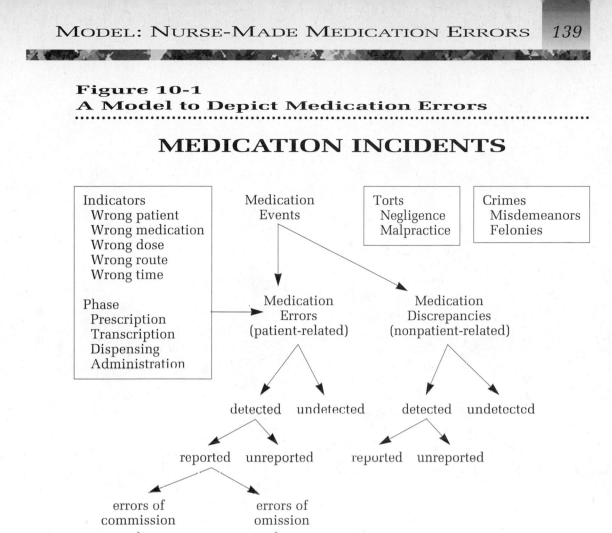

Indicators
  Wrong patient
  Wrong medication
  Wrong dose
  Wrong route
  Wrong time

Phase
  Prescription
  Transcription
  Dispensing
  Administration

Medication
Events

Torts
  Negligence
  Malpractice

Crimes
  Misdemeanors
  Felonies

Medication
Errors
(patient-related)

Medication
Discrepancies
(nonpatient-related)

detected   undetected   detected   undetected

reported   unreported   reported   unreported

errors of
commission

errors of
omission

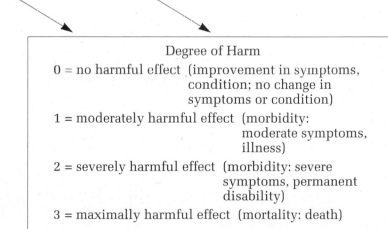

Degree of Harm

0 = no harmful effect (improvement in symptoms,
                        condition; no change in
                        symptoms or condition)

1 = moderately harmful effect (morbidity:
                                moderate symptoms,
                                illness)

2 = severely harmful effect (morbidity: severe
                              symptoms, permanent
                              disability)

3 = maximally harmful effect (mortality: death)

The consequences of medication errors can be described or scaled according to the degree of harm done to the patient:

- No harmful effect: Improvement in symptoms or condition, or no change in symptoms or condition.
- A moderately harmful effect: Some evidence of change in patient status (morbidity: moderate symptoms, illness).
- A severely harmful effect: Morbidity: severe symptoms, permanent disability.
- The maximally harmful effect: Death.

The model also includes indicators of medication errors that are frequently cited in the literature, among them, wrong dose, wrong drug, wrong time, and wrong route of administration. In addition, it specifies the phase of preparation or administration (prescription, transcription, dispensing, administration) when the error took place.

The model needs to be scrutinized carefully by nurses. Each time a medication error occurs, the model should be evaluated to determine if it is useful in classifying and describing the mistake. Furthermore, error rates are often reported with little description of the antecedent conditions, which may contribute to the actual error, or of the immediate and long-term results of the mistake, which may be monitored as a patient's status changes. One of the studies included in Appendixes employed the model as a guide for a questionnaire to elicit descriptions of actual medication errors. Future efforts at model development and testing could help to clarify the nature of medication errors and help health care providers to target their efforts to preventing and minimizing harm once errors occur.

REFERENCES

Faddis, M. O. (1939). Eliminating errors in medication. *American Journal of Nursing, 39*(11), 1217–1223.

Wolf, Z. R. (1986). *Nurses' work: The sacred and the profane.* Philadelphia: University of Pennsylvania Press.

Wolf, Z. R. (1989). Medication errors and nursing responsibility. *Holistic Nursing Practice, 4*(1), 8–17.

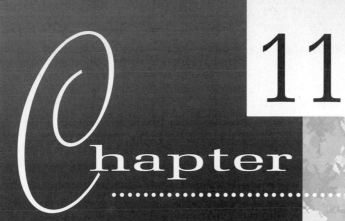

Chapter 11

Nurses' Mistakes at Work: An Essay

Often nurses know a great deal about the patients they care for. They meet family members and friends and are aware of personal histories. Nurses grow to understand the ways of their patients and see them against a rich context because of this understanding. As a result of this personal knowledge, nurses are very troubled when they make mistakes at work.

The medication-related mistakes that nurses make are at times more fateful than other occupational groups' mistakes. The possibility of the worst fate, the death of a patient following an error, frightens nurses and their teachers the most. This fear is connected implicitly to the principle of doing no harm. The special combination of knowledge and skill that nursing students, graduate nurses, and nurse orientees possess is monitored by nursing professors and staff development instructors. In addition, seasoned nurses, nurse managers, and nurse administrators serve as a peer review system. As teachers, they test, instruct, and observe the performance of those new to different aspects of medication administration. They ensure for a short time that few mistakes will be made and that no harm will be done.

Patients may suffer when medication errors are made. Often these patients never know of the error, since the clinical effects that result may not be present or recognizable to patients or their families. Patients, moreover, believe in the skills of nurses and trust them to carry out their work. Their faith is compromised when the risky business of nursing is evident in a medication error and a patient is harmed. And since patients have delegated their care to nurses, the risks, the failure, and the harm are shared.

E. C. Hughes, a sociologist, examined a common theme in work: mistakes and failures. He suggested that the more often a skill is demonstrated and the more skillful the practitioner is, the more likely is the event of a mistake at work. Seasoned nurses make mistakes, and those who make medication errors are startled and dismayed at these mistakes.

Hughes viewed occupations as collections of skills, some of them requiring more practice in order to attain perfect performance compared to others. Even though some nurses have attained considerable skill in medication administration, they still make mistakes.

Hughes also suggested that occupational groups recognize the probability of making an error during work and develop a "collective rationale" to keep up their courage in the face of this possibility. Many nurses assert that every nurse makes mistakes and find comfort in that generalization. Through another nurse's telling of a medication error story, a nurse who recently committed an error may take comfort and courage and be challenged to go on. Moreover, spreading the risk around to the collective of nurses who work on that unit or who were involved in the patient's care helps the individual nurse to deal with the mistake. The collective or corporate guilt is shared by the nurse most involved in the error and his or her colleagues. In this way, the guilt and responsibility are spread throughout the unit.

Nurses decide whether a medication error has occurred and then gauge the amount of harm done to the patient and the potential harm that may befall them. Other nurses, physicians, and pharmacists act as a decision-making group of professional colleagues when an error is known to a larger group. Whether the error is labeled as such rests on individual or group opinion of professionals. "The colleague-group will consider that it alone fully understands the technical contingencies, and that it should therefore be given the sole right to say when a mistake has been made. . . . This attitude may be extended to complete silence concerning mistakes of a member of the colleague group, because the very discussion before a larger audience may imply the right of the layman to make a judgment; and it is the right to make the judgment that is most jealously guarded" (Hughes, 1951). However, patients, family members, and friends may be very aware of the mistake.

Technology and science continue to produce medications to cure and stabilize patients and to prevent disease. The complexity of medication administration will increase as new products arrive and challenge nurses' knowledge and skill. And despite vigilance, medication errors will persist.

REFERENCE

Hughes, E. C. (1951). Mistakes at work. *Journal of Economics and Political Science, 17*, 320–327.

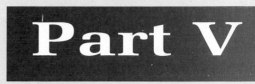

Part V

Appendixes

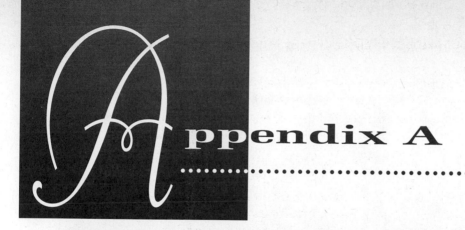

Appendix A

Effect of Three Teaching Methods on Nursing Staff's Knowledge of Medication Error Risk-Reduction Strategies

A Research Proposal

Elaine R. Volk
Rita S. Jablonski
Terry B. McGoldrick
Zane Robinson Wolf
Linda M. Dean
Eileen P. McKee

INTRODUCTION

When nurses administer medications, they are committed to uphold an ethical principle: to do good and avoid harm. Although they may not explicitly frame their practice in terms of this principle, they are nevertheless socialized to it in schools of nursing and at work, and they violate it when they make medication errors (Wolf, 1989). Fundamentals of nursing textbooks contain explicit reinforcements of the principle—for example, "When an error does occur, the nurse's first responsibility must be to the patient. The error needs to be reported immediately and measures taken to correct the error if it is indicated" (Kozier & Erb, 1979). Drug errors may be one of the most frequent mistakes nurses make; at times they result in lawsuits (Poteet, 1983; Springhouse Corp., 1992).

Medication errors are unintentional mistakes associated with drugs and intravenous solutions that involve patients and are made during the prescription, transcription, dispensing, and administration phases of drug preparation and distribution (Wolf, 1989). There are two types of medication errors: errors of omission and errors of commission. These mistakes at work, whether involving a nurse alone or in association with a physician or pharmacist, can jeopardize patient, provider, and institutional safety.

System-originated errors—for example, similar labeling of different drugs—can be corrected. But random errors—those that occur by chance and in no particular pattern—are difficult to eliminate (Elnicki & Schmitt, 1980). In spite of retrospective and prospective efforts by nurses, risk managers, and other hospital personnel, it may be impossible to prevent them. Nevertheless, nurses share the responsibility to reduce such errors.

The administrators of two nursing service organizations decided to target their efforts on a prospective program designed to reduce medication errors made by nursing personnel and the risks consequent to medication errors. They directed their work toward an educational intervention to affect staff nurses' knowledge of the risks related to medication errors. The study reported here compares the effects of three teaching strategies (videotape, instructional booklet, and lecture) on registered nurse (RN) and licensed practical nurse (LPN) knowledge of medication error risk-reduction strategies and then compares RN and LPN knowledge of medication error risk-reduction strategies (Wolf, 1989, 1992).

REVIEW OF THE LITERATURE

Nurses are keenly aware that they serve "as the final checkpoint in the system" for administering medications (Adams & Burleson, 1992, p. 951). They rely on personal and professional rituals, hospital procedures, action plans, and advice to prevent them from making errors (Kaplan, 1991; Keill & Johnson, 1993; Springhouse Corp., 1991; Wolf, 1986, 1992). At times, preventive strategies fail, leaving many distressed by their mistakes and searching for additional tactics to prevent future errors.

Since patient harm can result from medication errors, and harm is considered the worst-case scenario for hospital nursing practice, nurse administrators take the position that no errors are acceptable. However, this zero-tolerance standard may be impossible to realize (Manthey, 1989a) and may simply result in reducing the number of errors that are reported by nurses.

Health care institutions try to prevent medication errors by publishing preventive strategies in their policies and procedures manuals, and they introduce nursing staff to these standards of care during orientation sessions. Risk management departments in health care institutions also attempt to eliminate harm to patients, personnel, and the hospital by reducing the costs associated with unusual events or incidents, such as medication errors (Poteet, 1983).

Nurses have created rules and ritualistic checks to keep them from making medication errors. These serve to help nurses focus on the task at hand when surrounded by distractions. One of these guidelines is the "five rights" rule: the nurse must give the (1) right drug to the (2) right patient at the (3) right time in the (4) right dosage by the (5) right route (Hodgin, 1984; Ludwig-Beymer, Czurylo, Gattuso, Hennesscy & Ryan, 1990; Springhouse Corp., 1992; Sullivan, 1991). Another is the three-time checks (Ludwig-Beymer et al., 1990), which has been repeated in the nursing literature for nearly a century (Groff, 1896): "When you are about to measure a dose of medicine, look for your bottle, read the label, and then reach for it. As you raise the measuring glass to a level with your eye, look at the label again. Measure the medicine, and, as you return the bottle to its place, again read the label. Here are three chances to correct a possible error; always take advantage of them" (p. 638).

Nursing service organizations have developed point systems to evaluate medication errors, along with protocols to determine disciplinary actions (Cobb, 1990; Lowery, 1991) and severity indexes to determine actions to take following errors (Brandt, Deml, Gerke & Lee, 1988; Walters et al., 1992). These approaches ensure more uniform handling of medication errors and may positively influence the rate of reporting medication errors. More systematic classification and weighing of medication errors could increase awareness of causative factors among nurses and result in reduced error rates and more consistent follow-up. However, it is the opinion of some nurses that point systems might inhibit reporting of medication errors rather than serve to prevent errors.

Many nurses, after they make medication errors, feel guilty and may expect or desire some form of punishment or reparation as payment for their mistake (Wolf, 1989, 1992). Others fear punishment, which may vary from the "emotional pain of shame and guilt" (Manthey, 1989, p. 19) to more public forms of humiliation and termination from their jobs. Manthey (1989a) suggested that discipline and punishment are synonymous to nurses. However, the terms are not synonymous since punishment causes pain, whereas discipline maintains order. Subsequently, Manthey (1989b) proposed that nonpunitive responses to mistakes at work provide the wrongdoer with the opportunity to gain knowledge and skill and to revise attitudes about medication errors. One example of using education rather than punishment following a medication error is the EDMET (El Dorado Medication Error Tool) form (Cobb, 1990), which employs a point system to evaluate errors. The EDMET approach specifies counseling and education sessions. The education component includes a medication review class and a self-learning packet on medication administration procedures.

Providing corrective action that involves education may result in nurses' reporting more medication errors, since the action taken is no longer seen as punitive. McClure (1991) suggested that since human error can only be reduced, not eliminated, nursing needs to become more forgiving of these errors while demanding corrective action, especially when patient safety is threatened. An educational program could provide a more temperate approach to dealing with the nurse involved in a medication error and could serve to retain a competent practitioner for the hospital and the profession. A medication error does not automatically imply incompetence.

Ludwig-Beymer et al. (1990) investigated the effect of eliminating a medication test designed to measure nurses' knowledge of medication administration on the medication error rate. The investigators used incident reports to measure the rate of errors for two years over the same eight months and found that the overall number of medication errors decreased (3.5%); some errors increased (wrong patient, wrong dose, wrong time, wrong route, duplication of dose, and delay), and some decreased (wrong rate, wrong medication, omission, and allergy). These conclusions should be viewed with caution, since intervening variables not under the control of the investigators could have affected the decreased rate. Based on this study, it may not be advisable to eliminate the medication test given to nursing staff during orientation or annual mandatory in-service programs.

In a computer-simulated study aimed at describing clinical decision making of 142 critical care nurses, Henry (1991) found that medication errors were the cause of death in 87 percent of the simulations. Types of medication errors resulting in simulated patient death included administering a medication that was contraindicated, administering a medication to which the patient was allergic, and medication overdose. Boggs, Brown-Molnar, and DeLapp (1988) investigated nurses' knowledge of three commonly prescribed drugs, differences in specific types of nurses' drug knowledge, and the relationship between level of knowledge and educational or experiential background. Using a 36-item test and a demographic questionnaire, the investigators determined that respondents overall had an inadequate level of knowledge, with an identifiable difference in knowledge between BSN- and LPN-prepared nursing staff. Practical experience was not related to drug knowledge, since nurse administrators, managers, and public health nurses had more knowledge than the nurses responsible for drug administration. The investigators recommended continuing the practice of administering examinations to test nurses' drug knowledge during orientation programs, as well as ongoing and regular programs for nurses who administer medications. They questioned the advisability of assigning medication administration to nurses with limited educational preparation, such as LPNs, because they demonstrated consistently low scores on the test. Few studies, however, have addressed differences between RN and LPN performance on medication administration tests of knowledge. Furthermore, no studies were located that compared knowledge of medication administration or error rates among full-time nurses, graduate nurses, and agency nurses.

Cohen (1990) created a test based on actual medication errors to help nurses increase their knowledge of risks associated with medication errors. The self-test was presented as a way to test personal knowledge, not as a research study. In contrast, the test in Ludwig-Beymer et al. (1990) study was composed of dosage calculation problems and general application questions to test safe practice in this area. Similarly, Bindler and Bayne (1991) investigated 110 RNs' medication calculation ability using a 20-item test. The error rate was highest for intravenous calculation problems and next for oral and intramuscular/subcutaneous problems. Nurses' error rates increased when more than one calculation was involved in a problem and when milligram-to-grain conversions were required. Blais and Bath (1992) also tested drug calculation skills of 66 nursing students using a 20-item test. Conceptual errors (set-up and form) were the most frequent (33 percent) calculation mistakes, followed by mathematical (19 percent) and measurement errors (13 percent). No studies were located investigating the use of a teaching intervention aimed at increasing nurses' knowledge of the risks associated with medication errors and strategies to prevent errors and risks and patient harm following errors.

Nurses' mistakes, similar to those of pharmacists and physicians, can be more harmful than those of other occupations because of the human, personal care aspects of their occupation. When a medication error occurs, not only personal, but departmental and institutional risks are evident, as are the risk-dispersing devices used by nurses. As the mistake unfolds, nurses put into use the "collective rationale which they whistle to one another to keep up their courage" (Hughes, 1951, p. 321). Often the mistake is "owned" in a corporate sense by the nurses directly and indirectly involved in the medication error (Wolf, 1986).

Wolf (1989) constructed a model to explain risks, types, and patient consequences of nurse-made medication errors. The model was generated from ethnographic study of nursing rituals (Wolf, 1986), since nurse informants in the study classified types and variations in the types of medication errors, and from the literature reviewed for an article on medication errors (Wolf, 1989). It was recently revised as a result of other studies on medication errors; these studies used phenomenological, focus group, and story-telling methods (Wolf, 1992). (See Figure 10–1.) This model was used along with related literature to guide the content of the items on a test of knowledge aimed at preventing medication errors and managing the risks associated with them.

THEORETICAL FRAMEWORK

Knowles's (1980) adult learning theory (ALT) provides the theoretical framework for this study. Knowles's concept of andragogy, or teaching that is geared to adults, spans many categories of behaviorist learning theory. ALT acknowledges the value of reinforcement (Skinner, 1969) and social learning principles (Bandura, 1974). Andragogical approaches to adult learning emphasize self-determination, self-assessment, and involvement of the whole person in the learning process. Adult learners move from dependent to self-directed learning. They draw from an accumulation of experiences as a potential resource for their own and other learners' acquisition of knowledge and skills. In ALT, the emphasis is placed on the practical application of learning using strategies to help the learner link conceptual formulations and practical needs to educational objectives. Furthermore, ALT is problem focused.

Self-directed learning is preferred by adult learners in general (Estrine, 1975; Knowles, 1980; Tough, 1978), including health care professionals (Emblem & Gray, 1989; Goldrick, 1989; McNaull, Bel & and Clipp, 1992; Santopietro, 1980). Programmed instruction and self-learning modules are examples of self-directed learning strategies and provide the learner with immediate feedback for mastery of tasks (Mast & Van Atta, 1986). In this study, the instructional booklet is an example of an approach to self-directed learning.

METHODS

The medication error teaching method study will be implemented using a pretest/posttest design. Male and female nursing staff from two nursing service organizations will be requested to participate in the study. RNs and LPNs will be obtained by a convenience sampling technique. Only RNs and LPNs who administer medications will constitute the study sample. Subjects will be randomly assigned to the videotape (N = 50), instructional booklet (N = 50), or lecture (N = 50) group. The effect of the teaching interventions will be compared using posttest scores (appendix D).

Instrumentation

A 38-item test—21 true-false, 3 matching, and 5 multiple-choice items and 9 calculation problems—will be administered to videotape, instructional booklet, and lecture group subjects. Test items were generated from a thorough literature review on risk-reduction strategies in order to support the test's content validity. Calculation problems were written to test skill in drug dosage computation. In addition, the first version of the test was critiqued by a chief nurse executive, a risk-reduction officer, a pharmacist, a nurse quality assurance coordinator, a director of nursing, a nurse manager, and three staff nurses. They served as an expert panel and judged the content validity and clarity of test items. One master's-prepared and one doctoral-prepared nurse educator judged the congruence of the test items with the teaching plan. Test items were revised and eliminated following these reviews. The test was administered to a pilot group of ten nurses, roughly comparable to the population to be in the sample. Test-retest reliability was established using the same initial pilot group of ten RNs; the test was relatively stable over a 2-week interval ($r = .40$, $p = .000$). The test was revised; one item was eliminated, and three items were revised. Test-retest reliability was calculated again on nine RNs; the test was stable over a 1-week interval ($r = .92$, $p = .000$). The revised test was administered to eight RNs; item difficulty scores ranged from .37 (most difficult item) to 1.0 (least difficult item).

Next, the test was revised and administered to ten RNs to establish test-retest reliability; the test was stable ($r = .75$, $p = .03$) following a 5-hour interval. Test difficulty was calculated (1/2 total number of items: $45/2 = 22.5$); the mean of the test for ten RNs was 36.1. At this time, item discrimination (Net $D = R_u - R_l/N_u$) was calculated for all 45 items of the test. Based on validity coefficients, the test was again revised; several items were edited and eliminated, leaving 41 items on the test. The revised test was administered to ten RNs attending an RN-BSN program. Test difficulty and item discrimination were again calculated. Items were revised and deleted, and additional dosage calculation problems were added. Next, the test was administered to 15 RNs and LPNs comparable to the study population; it was revised again based on item discrimination coefficients (Marshall & Hales, 1971).

The 41-item test was administered to 45 nurses who were comparable to the study population. Twenty-nine RNS and 16 LPNs completed this version. Test difficulty was 32. Item discrimination (Net $D = R_u - R_l/N_u$) was calculated for all 41 items of the test; index of item difficulty ($D = R/N$) was also calculated. Selected items were revised, added, or deleted from the test, based on these coefficients.

Procedures for Data Collection

Nursing staff will be approached during regularly scheduled educational offerings and committee meetings. They will be invited to consent to participate in the study. Group membership will be determined by random assignment to videotape, instructional booklet, or lecture conditions. Following the pretest, each group will be instructed; the posttest will next be administered.

DATA ANALYSIS

SPSS-x, a statistical package, will be used for data analysis. Descriptive statistics on demographic characteristics of subjects and on test items will also be computed. Posttest scores will be analyzed using ANOVA on group scores. A Tukey test will also be calculated. RN and LPN pretest scores will be compared using a t-test.

REFERENCES

Adams, T. D., & Burleson, K. W. (1992, June). Continuous quality improvement in a medication error reporting system. *P&T*, 943–951.

Bandura, A. (1974). Self-efficacy mechanism in human aging. *American Psychologist, 37*(2), 122–147.

Bindler, R., & Bayne, T. (1991). Medication calculation ability of registered nurses. *Image, 23*(4), 221–224.

Blais, K., & Bath, J. G. (1992). Drug calculation errors of baccalaureate nursing students. *Nurse Educator, 17*(1), 12–15.

Boggs, P., Brown-Molnar, C. S., & DeLapp, T. D. (1988). Nurses' drug knowledge. *Western Journal of Nursing Research, 10*(1), 84-93.

Brandt, M., Deml, M., Gerke, M. L., & Lee, E. H. (1988). A severity index for medication errors. *Nursing Management, 19*(8), 80i–80p.

Cobb, M. D. (1990, March). Dealing fairly with medication errors. *Nursing '90,* pp. 42–43.

Cohen, M. R. (1990). Medication errors. *Nursing '90, 20*(3), 23–24.

Elnicki, R. A., & Schmitt, J. P. (1980). Contributions of patient and hospital characteristics to adverse incidents. *Health Services Research, 15,* 398–414.

Emblem, J., & Gray, G. (1989). Comparison of nurses' self-directed learning activities. *Journal of Continuing Education in Nursing, 21*(2), 56–61.

Estrine, L. (1975). The effectiveness of linear versus branching programmed instuctional methods in adult cognitive learning. *Dissertation Abstracts International, 36,* 1378A.

Goldrick, B. A. (1989). Programmed instruction revisited: A solution to infection control inservice education. *Journal of Continuing Education in Nursing, 20*(5), 222–227.

Groff, J. (1896). Hand-book of materia medica for trained nurses. *Trained Nurse, 16,* 635–640.

Henry, S. B. (1991). Clinical decision making of critical care nurses managing computer-simulated tachydysrhythmias. *Heart and Lung, 20*(5), 469–477.

Hodgin, L. (1984). Sarnia General develops medication error report. *Dimensions in Health Service, 61*(3), 25–43.

Hughes, E. C. (1951). Mistakes at work. *Journal of Economics and Political Science, 17*, 320–327.

Kaplan, M. J. (1991). Experiences of registered nurses and physicians with making medication errors. Unpublished master's thesis, La Salle University, Philadelphia, PA.

Keill, P., & Johnson, T. (1993). Shifting gears: Improving delivery of medications. *Journal of Nursing Quality Assurance, 7*(2), 24–33.

Knowles, M. S. (1980). *The modern practice of adult education: From pedagogy to andragogy* (2d ed.). New York: Adult Education Co.

Kozier, B., & Erb, G. L. (1979). *Fundamentals of nursing.* Menlo Park, CA: Addison-Wesley.

Lowery, K. (1991). *Medication error prevention through trending and reporting of errors.* Grand View Hospital, Quality Assurance Department, Grand View, PA.

Ludwig-Beymer, P., Czurylo, K. T., Gattuso, M. C., Hennessy, K. A., & Ryan, C. J. (1990). The effect of testing on the reported incidence of medication errors in a medical center. *Journal of Continuing Education in Nursing, 21*(1), 11–17.

McClure, M. L. (1991). Human error—A professional dilemma. *Journal of Professional Nursing, 7*(4), 207.

McNaull, F., Belyea, M., & Clipp, E. (1992). A comparison of educational methods to enhance nursing performance in pain assessment. *Journal of Continuing Education in Nursing, 23*(6), 267–271.

Manthey, M. (1989a, October). Discipline without punishment—Part I. *Nursing Management*, p. 19.

Manthey, M. (1989b, November). Discipline without punishment—Part II. *Nursing Management,* p. 23.

Marshall, J. C., & Hales, L. W. (1971). *Classroom test construction.* Reading, MA: Addison-Wesley.

Mast, M., & Van Atta, M. J. (1986). Applying adult learning principles in instructional module design. *Nurse Educator, 11*(1), 35–39.

Poteet, G. W. (1983). Risk management and nursing. *Nursing Clinics of North America, 18*(3), 457–465.

Santopietro, M. (1980). Effectiveness of self-instructional module in human sexuality counseling. *Nursing Research, 29*, 14–19.

Skinner, B. F. (1969). *Contingencies of reinforcement.* New York: Appleton-Century-Crofts.

Springhouse Corp. (1991). *Nurses' book of advice.* Springhouse, PA: Author.

Springhouse Corp. (1992). *Nurse's handbook of law and ethics.* Springhouse, PA: Author.

Sullivan, G. H. (1991). Five "rights" equal 0 errors. *RN, 54*(6), 65–66, 68.

Tough, A. (1978). Major learning efforts: Recent research and future dimensions. *Adult Education, 28*, 250–263.

Walters, J. A., Puetz, C., Sala, S. M., Hanson, K., Beder, L., Maxon, P., & Crucius, L. (1992). Developing and implementing a tool to measure severity of medication errors. *Journal of Nursing Care Quality, 6*(4), 33–43.

Wolf, Z. R. (1986). *Nurses' work: The sacred and the profane.* Philadelphia: University of Pennsylvania Press.

Wolf, Z. R. (1989). Medication errors and nursing responsibility. *Holistic Nursing Practice, 4*(1), 8–17.

Wolf, Z. R. (1992). *Nurses' experiences making medication errors.* Unpublished manuscript.

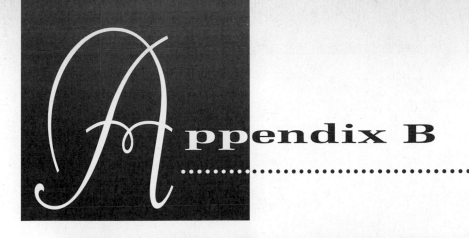

Appendix B

Medication Error Risk-Reduction Teaching Plan

The purpose of the Medication Error Risk-Reduction Teaching Plan (Appendix B) is to organize pertinent information on how to avoid making medication errors and to minimize the effects of errors after they are made. The teaching plan was used on the study cited in Appendix A to organize the content for a videotape, lecture, and instructional booklet (Appendix C).

Objective	Content	Strategies

	I. Safe patient care
	  A. Professional commitment
	  B. Quality patient care and professional practice
	    1. Accountability
	    2. Responsibility
		Lecture/discussion

■ Define a medication error
 	
■ Compare different types of medication error/incidents
 	
■ Weigh the severity of different types of medication errors
 	
■ Give examples of different types of medication errors
	II. Medication error
	  A. Definition
	  B. Model
	    1. Errors of omission
	      a. Examples
	    2. Errors of commission
	      a. Examples
	    3. Patient harm
	      a. Degree
	  C. Indicators
		Handout: Model

Objective	Content	Strategies

■ Describe the functions of rules, rituals, and policies and procedures in relation to preventing medication errors	III. Prevention
	  A. Rules
	    1. Nursing lore
	    2. Fundamentals or foundations courses
	      a. Socialization
	  B. Rituals
	    1. Personal
	    2. Professional
	  C. Policy and procedure manuals
	    1. Standards of practice
	    2. Legal implications
	      a. Nurse practice acts
	    3. Definitions of medication error
	    4. Expected behaviors and sequence of events
	      a. Legal implications of policies and procedures
	    1. Reporting medication errors
	    2. Verbal orders
		Questions/answers

■ Explain the responsibilities of risk management staff, hospital administrators, nurse managers, quality assurance coordinators, and staff nurses in relation to patient safety	IV. Administrative responsibilities: Patient safety and quality patient care
	  A. Counseling, education, termination
	  B. Corporation, hospital, department, unit, nurse, patient
	    1. Liability
	    2. Organizational chart
	  C. Attitudes: Responsibility and carelessness	

■ Evaluate the impact of a serious medication error on all parts of the institution	V. Types of risks
	  A. Psychological, physical, social, legal, ethical, moral, economic
	  B. Impact of risks on different parts of the system: personal (patient and employee), unit, departmental, hospital, corporation	

Objective	Content	Strategies

	VI. Risk reduction
	A. Risk management department
	  1. Scope of responsibility
	  2. Chain of reporting
	    a. Staff appraisal of error rate by unit
	B. Containing random, system, and human errors: Illusions and realities
	C. Liability insurance	

▪ List the methods used to track medication errors	VII. Medication error tracking systems
	A. Reported errors
	B. Incident reports
	C. Quality assurance coordinator for nursing
	  1. Monitoring errors on a unit level
	D. Risk manager and medication error rate
	  1. Monitoring hospital-wide medication error incidence rates
	  2. Legal implications	

▪ Describe actions and other strategies employed to reduce the risk of medication errors	VIII. Strategies to reduce risk of medication errors
	A. Nurse strategies
	  1. Follow rules passed down in nursing: three-times check and five rights
	  2. Read and follow procedure on medication administration
		Lecture/discussion

Objective	Content	Strategies

3. Use personal rituals
   a. Differentiation between unsafe practices and rituals
4. Follow accepted routines
   a. Prescribed time and accepted time range to administer drugs on time
5. Keep current with new pharmaceuticals
6. Periodic refresher of drug and solution calculations
   a. Problem setup/form
   b. Mathematics
   c. Procedures for conversion between two measurement systems
7. Go to clinical specialist, pharmacist, physician, formulary, and textbooks for expert knowledge
8. Question hospital personnel, including other nurses, physicians, pharmacists
   a. Resolve question about unfamiliar drugs
9. Listen to the patient
10. "When in doubt, don't"
11. Use clinical judgment, which is shaped by knowledge about the patient (contraindication to patient's condition)
12. Know the patient from a holistic view
13. Carefully transcribe and check transcriptions
14. Read labels carefully
    a. Lack of standardization of labels among manufacturers

Objective	Content	Strategies
	15. Be aware of ambiguous drug names and orders (ambiguous and atypical)	
	16. Question sudden and excessive increases in medication dosage and frequency of administration	
	17. Be careful of patient with hypersensitivity; administer newly ordered drugs cautiously a. Cross-sensitivity	
	18. Check for drug interactions and potentiation effects	
	19. Check if it is appropriate to check a specific medication for oral or GI tube route	
	20. Check look-alike and sound-alike drug names	
	21. Check potassium chloride labels carefully	
	22. Do not administer medication poured by another nurse, pharmacist, physician a. "Reality" check	
	23. Be aware of risks noted in related literature a. Medication time scheduled during shift report b. Medication times scheduled frequently during 24-hour day c. Nurse working first or second day back to work after time off d. Long response time after medication ordered e. Defective packaging f. Prescription problems: no strength, time, directions, etc. specified g. New medication order	

Objective	Content	Strategies
	h. Older patients involved in medication errors more than younger patients i. Most medication errors occur between 6 A.M. and 12 P.M. j. Greater number of medications nurse administers, the greater chance of error	

▪ Explain objective approaches to documenting medication errors	IX. Medication error documentation
	A. Identify an incident "commander"
	B. Take action
	C. Notify charge nurse, nurse manager, attending physician, pharmacy, and other appropriate departments
	  1. Follow policy and avoid poor advice
	D. Document action
	  1. Incident report, nurses' notes, medication administration record
	E. Complete incident report as soon as possible after discovery
	  1. State facts, not subjective opinion
	F. Risk manager tracks patient's progress	

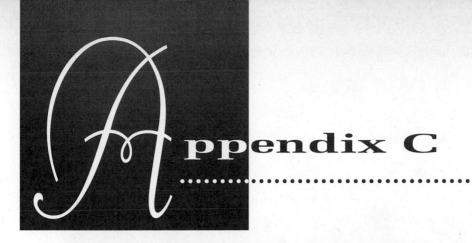

Appendix C

Programmed Instruction for Reduction of Medication Errors

The Programmed Instruction for Reduction of Medication Errors was created as a self-paced learning booklet for staff nurses enrolled as subjects in the study included in Appendix A. The booklet was used as one of three teaching strategies in a study completed during 1993. Three interventions where compared in relation to nurses' knowledge scores: the programmed instruction, a lecture, and a videotape. The content of the booklet was guided by the teaching plan included in Appendix B.

OBJECTIVES

After completing this module, participants will be able to:

1. Define a medication error.
2. Compare different types of medication errors/incidents.
3. Give examples of different types of medication errors/incidents.
4. Weigh the severity of different types of medication errors.
5. Explain the responsibilities of risk management, hospital administrators, nurse managers, quality assurance coordinators, and staff nurses in relation to patient safety.
6. Describe the functions of rules, rituals, and policies and procedures in relation to preventing medication errors.
7. Evaluate the impact of a serious medication error on all parts of the institution.
8. List the methods used to track medication errors.

Prepared with the help of Rita Seeger Jablonski.

9. Explain objective approaches to documenting medication errors.
10. Describe actions and other strategies employed to reduce the risk of medication errors.

Directions: Read the following sections carefully. Do all of the exercises that follow certain sections. You can write your answer in the spaces provided. The correct answers are given immediately after each exercise. Do not proceed to the next sections until you are comfortable with the content covered in the preceding sections.

DEFINITION OF MEDICATION ERROR

A medication error is defined as a mistake that is made at work when nurses administer drugs ordered by physicians and dispensed by pharmacists. Medication errors are unintentional mistakes in the prescription, transcription, dispensing, and administration of drugs and intravenous solutions. The patient receives a medication incorrectly or fails to receive it.

There are two types of errors:

- *Error of omission:* An incident in which a patient does not receive a prescribed drug because the nurse unintentionally failed to give a prescribed drug.

- *Error of commission*: A nurse inadvertently gives a patient a drug that was not prescribed or an excessive dose of a prescribed medication.

Other Medication Incidents

Not all incidents involving medications and patients fit neatly into the categories of omission and commission. Some incidents are purposeful acts designed to cause patient harm or designed to divert medication. Whereas most unintentional medication incidents involved in lawsuits are labeled negligence, purposeful acts may be classified as felonies. For example, a nurse addicted to morphine may steal the drug and give the patient saline injections. In another example, a nurse may intentionally give patients Pavulon (pancuronium bromide) to paralyze them and next play hero by resuscitating them. There have been deaths reported because of intentional acts involving medications.

The nurses who intentionally perform such acts may be arrested and tried in courts of law.

DEGREES OF HARM

Different degrees of harm can occur to patients when errors of omission or errors of commission are made. For example, two patients allergic to penicillin receive this drug. One patient experiences a mild rash, which fades after the drug is discontinued. The other patient experiences acute respiratory failure and requires mechanical ventilation. Both patients received the incorrect drug, and both suffered, but the second patient's ordeal was worse. He experienced a greater degree of harm than the first.

When discussing the degree of harm incurred from a medication incident, it is useful to think of harm as a continuum. Obviously, death is the worst harm possible. Next is the presence of symptoms. As demonstrated by the example, the types of symptom also affect the degree of harm suffered by the patient. At times, there are no noticeable results following a medication error. On occasion, the patient's condition might actually improve as a result of the error. But regardless of the degree of harm suffered by the patient, a medication error is still a medication error.

Exercise 1

For each sentence below, indicate whether the situation is an error of omission (EO), an error of commission (EC), or a criminal act (CA).

1. _____ Nurse forgets to administer the 4 PM dose of intravenous vancomycin.

2. _____ Nurse switches parenteral morphine with saline; gives patient a saline injection, but keeps morphine for himself.

3. _____ Nurse administers long-acting insulin instead of short-acting insulin.

Answers: 1. EO   2. CA   3. EC

RECOGNIZING A MEDICATION ERROR

Several facts lead nurses to conclude that a medication error has been made. Often-cited indicators, or signs, include: wrong patient, wrong medication, wrong dose, wrong time, wrong route of administration, and wrong rate of administration.

Exercise 2

Identify the indicator (wrong patient, wrong medication, wrong dose, wrong time, or wrong route) for each medication error.

1. A patient receives 12.5 mg of digoxin instead of 0.125 mg.
    _____

2. Jack Smith receives John Smith's oral hypoglycemic agent.
    _____

3. Intravenous heparin infuses at a rate of 80 cc/hr instead of the prescribed 42 cc/hr. _____

4. Mrs. Slokum receives her antibiotic at 6 PM; it was ordered for 6 AM, 2 PM, and 10 PM. _____

5. Mr. McDade received his subcutaneous heparin as an intra-muscular injection. _____

6. While giving out her medications, Nurse Walsh gives the patient chewable dilantin 50 mg instead of the sustained-release dilantin that was ordered. _____

Answers: 1. Wrong dose   2. Wrong patient   3. Wrong rate
         4. Wrong time   5. Wrong route   6. Wrong medication

GRAY AREAS

The definition of a medication error is confounded by many gray areas, such as the one nurses describe as the "magic hour." In this case, an error may technically have occurred, yet the nurses decide not to label it as one or not to treat it as one.

For example, an iron supplement is ordered at 10 AM, 2 PM, and 6 PM. The patient has a 9:30 appointment in the physical therapy department, so the nurses give the medication at 8 AM, not 10 AM. Because it is iron, the nurses think that it makes sense to give it with breakfast. But the nurses do not ask the physician to write the order that way, nor do they write the actual time that the medication was given in the medication administration record.

This kind of circumstance is common, and deviation from the prescription does not constitute an error in the eyes of most nurses. However, it is difficult to explain the rules to nursing students and graduate nurses when the extenuating circumstances of nursing practice encourage seasoned nurses to bend rules. The nurses who were involved in a situation similar to the previous one with the iron supplement did not violate anything in terms of patient safety; in fact, they added their own good judgment to a situation that the physician was unaware of or had not thought through carefully. The nurses, in

Exercise 3

Indicate whether the following statements are true or false.

1. _____ Because iron, vitamins, and antacids are over-the-counter medications, nurses can give them at times other than when they are actually ordered.

2. _____ In order to avoid making a medication error, the nurse should have a physician rewrite a medication order when patient or unit activities prevent that medication from being given at the prescribed time.

Answers: 1. False   2. True

turn, may not feel obligated to fill out an incident report because, in their eyes, no error occurred. On the other hand, to bend the rules day after day is not sensible. Good judgment requires speaking with the physician and getting the order and the situation changed.

POLICIES AND PROCEDURES

Even though hospitals have policy and procedures manuals that detail the rules governing medication administration, nurses do not often read them. Instead, nurses tend to formulate their own private rules as to exactly what constitutes a medication error. For example, the policy and procedures manual may say that a nurse can give a medication 30 minutes before and 30 minutes after the time that it is ordered. While this hour is aimed at by most nurses, the reality of the clinical situation dictates that this is often not possible. In this scenario, the nurse is responsible for ten patients, five of whom are to receive insulin at 8 AM. Change-of-shift report starts at 7:30 AM and ends about 8:15 AM. How realistic is it to think that the nurse could administer the five insulin injections in 15 minutes? It is difficult to adhere to the time limits set forth in a medication administration procedure because different patient units have different time constraints and patient care issues. Thus, it would make sense for the nurses facing that particular situation to change the time that insulins are routinely administered.

Many nurses make their own decision about medication errors. They use their own personal definitions of medication errors. They might give the wrong drug but decide it is not a medication that could cause the patient harm. Their definition is based on the presence or absence of harm witnessed in the patient or anticipated to occur. One example of this scenario happens when a nurse forgets to give digoxin; this is considered a serious problem. On the other hand, forgetting to give Tagamet (cimetidine) is not considered to be such a problem. Although the patient might suffer from not getting the Tagamet, a nurse might not consider the omission to be serious.

In addition, nurses need to be aware that policies and procedures are standards of practice. For example, lawyers involved in a malpractice suit always scrutinize the policy and procedures of the hospital and would point out the discrepancies between the standard and the medication error incident if a patient received insulin too late and patient harm resulted. In both of these cases, the nurses' working definition of medication error violates policy and procedure.

Exercise 4

Indicate whether the following statements are true or false.

1. _____ Clinical reality, not accepted policy and procedures, dictates whether a nurse made a true medication error.

2. _____ When deciding to label a medication event as an error, the nurse needs to take into consideration patient harm.

3. _____ In order to prevent future medication errors, nurses need to evaluate whether their clinical practice supports accepted hospital standards of care.

Answers: 1. False   2. False   3. True

REPORTING THE ERROR

Nurses admit that they respond to medication errors in certain situations by not "ratting" on one another and may limit writing incident reports to only the most blatant errors. In contrast, others write incident reports frequently. Nurses equate the reporting of a medication error with an admission that they are not doing a good job or that good nursing practice is error-free practice. However, by definition, an error has taken place regardless of whether the nurse admits it. It happened in spite of the fact that a nurse failed to disclose it. When nurses admit that a mistake happened, that something has gone wrong, they acknowledge the warning that the mistake represents and try to improve care, based on this warning.

It is good advice to notify the charge nurse and the nurse manager about a medication error as soon as possible. The physician should be called immediately. At times the pharmacy should be notified so that pharmacists are alerted to the problem. Other departments, such as risk management, should be also notified. It may not be the best idea to inform some nurses who are not as seasoned as others about a medication error. The advice that some nurses give may be ill considered.

It may not be the best idea to assign the nurse who made the medication error to the involved patient, especially in the case of a patient who suffers harm. Some nurses may be so troubled by the error that they lose their clinical objectivity.

DOCUMENTING THE ERROR

Hospital policy and procedures manuals give directions to nurses, physicians, and pharmacists on how and to whom to report medication errors. All hospitals use incident reports and publish policies directing nurses and physicians about their responsibility. When they report a medication error, nurses have to be cautious about what they write about the mistake in hospital records. Nurses need to document what occurred in a factual manner without placing blame or adding value judgment. Nurses should be certain to address the problem with specific nursing interventions indicating that the patient is being monitored and cared for. It should be evident that the patient's vital signs are measured and recorded. Failing to document the fact that a nurse acted after the error and in response to the error suggests that the nursing staff did not acknowledge that the medication error took place. If it appears that the error was ignored or as if it never happened, nurses and others appear even more negligent about their care of the patient. All personnel who were notified of the error should be named in the chart. For example, nurses often write "MD notified," instead of recording, "Dr. Rubenstein notified." Nurses also need to document what is being done to monitor the patient and assess the patient for any possible complications.

In addition to the patient's chart, an incident report should be filled out. Ideally, the report is written by the nurse discovering the error. Again, the writer must document what actually happened without filling in opinion or conjecture. However, the nurse should never document in the patient chart that an incident report was filled out. This makes the incident report discoverable in a court of law.

Correct documentation on the chart and in the incident report is very important. First, the hospital needs to protect the patient, and second, the hospital needs evidence that action was taken in case of future lawsuits. It is generally accepted that if nurses and others try to cover these mistakes up, delay in taking action to correct them, or take action yet forget to document the interventions, many problems arise. In addition, the medication administration record includes documentation that a medication was not given or that another one was.

Exercise 5

Read the following paragraph and answer the questions.

While administering 6 PM medications, Dan Stefanopolus, RN, realizes that the 2 PM intravenous antibiotic for his patient was hung but never actually infused.

1. The first thing Dan should do is
   a. write an incident report.
   b. call the physician and let her know.
   c. give the missed antibiotic and then call the physician.

2. Dan documents the incident in his notes. He writes:
   a. "2 PM vancomycin found hanging but not infusing at 6 PM. I called the physician, Dr. Linda Suarez. She asked that I continue to give the antibiotic on its original schedule. The next dose is 10 PM tonight."
   b. "At 6 PM, I noticed that the 2 PM vancomycin was hanging but not infusing. The day nurse, Clare Jones, forgot to open up the clamp. I called Dr. Linda Suarez, who asked that I continue to give the antibiotic on its original schedule. The next dose is 10 PM tonight."
   c. "2 PM vancomycin found hanging but not infusing at 6 PM. I called the physician, Dr. Linda Suarez. She asked that I continue to give the antibiotic on its original schedule. The next dose will be given at 10 PM tonight. Incident report filed."

Answers: 1. b   2. a

CONSEQUENCES OF MEDICATION ERRORS

There are psychological risks to all involved in the error. When patients are hurt, the emotional repercussions can be devastating. There are social and economic harms as well. When patients remain in the hospital longer because of a medication error, they are separated from their family, and the family loses income if a breadwinner does not come home when expected.

In the case of other repercussions, colleagues may no longer trust the nurse who made the error. Distrust increases among fellow nurses if one of their co-workers continues to make medication errors. Also, a nursing unit may get a bad reputation. The news of the high error rates spreads rapidly through a hospital. There are costs for additional medications, nursing care hours, equipment, and supplies following certain medication errors.

Furthermore, legal costs incurred by suits tax the hospital and the plaintiff. The reputation of the hospital may suffer since it may be seen by the public as an unsafe place.

Exercise 6

Choose the best answer.

1. When a medication error occurs, who bears the consequences?
   a. The patient
   b. The nurse who committed the error
   c. The family of the patient
   d. All of the above

2. The cost of a medication error
   a. Can be easily measured in dollars and cents.
   b. Is difficult to determine because it entails monetary expenditures as well as human suffering.
   c. Is usually borne by the patient.
   d. Is written off as a loss at the end of the fiscal year.

Answers: 1. d   2. b

ROLE OF RISK MANAGEMENT

The risk management department surveys risks to the hospital and tries to contain such risks. Risk managers scrutinize the evidence and are removed from the people directly involved in the mistakes. They remain objective as they track problems over time. They try to help the individuals who are in more direct contact with the nurses who made the medication errors. The fact that the risk management department reports directly to the chief executive officer of the hospital underscores the seriousness of its charge.

PREVENTING MEDICATION ERRORS

Zero-Tolerance Rule

Hospital administrators subscribe to a zero-tolerance rule: the expectation that medication errors should not occur at all. They take this position out of fear of harming patients and concern for the liability issues that follow. But the zero-tolerance rule is violated often, since it is a human tendency to make mistakes. Thus, the rule may be unrealistic.

System Errors

The only errors that administrators may be successful with are systems errors: mistakes that occur because of a fundamental problem within a structure or entity. For example, if nurses notice that errors result during the transcription phase of medication administration, they can work to eliminate the problems in that particular part of the system. Another example of a systems problem that often results in medication errors is the problem of similar color or size labels on different intravenous medications.

Often systems errors can be addressed. In the second example given above, different manufacturers need to standardize labels on the same drugs. Nurses, pharmacists, and administrators need to be very alert to any kind of systems problem.

Random Errors

Random errors occur because of human mistakes, not systems problems. For example, a nurse mistakenly administers hydromorphone hydrochloride (Dilaudid) instead of morphine (morphine sulfate). It may be difficult or even impossible to eliminate these errors entirely. Strategies to reduce the chance of making random errors are discussed in a later section of this module.

Verbal Orders

Verbal orders given by a physician to a nurse that include a medication prescription can result in medication errors. Nurse administrators are very sensitive to the problems associated with verbal orders involving medications. According to nurses, physicians might give verbal orders over the telephone or in person and then later deny that they gave the order. In this situation, it is especially important to follow policy and procedure. Nurses get another nurse to witness the order, or both listen to the order at the same time. They also repeat the order twice and ask physicians to confirm its correctness. Physicians are expected to sign the order as soon as they come to the hospital, within 24 hours of the dated, timed order. Nurses do not appreciate taking verbal orders unless it is an emergency. However, they know that extenuating situations arise, since a resident physician often covers many patients at night or an attending physician could be scrubbed in for surgery.

Patient Alert

Nurses acknowledge that patients may be the first to alert them to a problem. If nurses are wise, they will not push their personal opinion on the patient or insist that they are right. There have been instances in which nurses have insisted and have ended up making a medication error. One rule that has served some nurses in this situation is the advice, "When in doubt, don't." The patient's uncertainty should plant uncertainty in the mind of the nurse.

Clinical Judgment

The clinical judgment of nurses might influence them to decide that giving a medication, even though it was ordered by a physician, could be considered an error. For example, a patient's condition gradually deteriorates. His kidneys are failing, and he is unable to excrete a medication that he has been receiving for some time. As nurses begin to become aware of this, they must stop administering the medication and rapidly notify the physician of their suspicions.

Errors During Transcription

Another opportunity for medication errors is present during transcription from the physician's order sheet to the medication administration record and pharmacy slips. The physician writes the medication order, and the medical clerk or the nurse transcribes the order and signs it off. The unit clerk's transcription is checked by the registered nurse. The next checkpoint takes place when the night nurse performs the

24-hour check. In addition, the nurse who prepared the medication for administration has the opportunity to check the transcription. Because of the flurry of activity of a busy patient unit, mistakes can be over-looked in spite of these checks.

Exercise 7

Indicate whether each statement is true or false.

1. _____ The zero-tolerance rule is a realistic expectation in regard to medication errors.

2. _____ Systems errors are easier to correct than random errors.

3. _____ When nurses accept verbal orders, they increase their risk of being involved in a medication error.

4. _____ It is a good idea to give a patient medication even after he or she has voiced concerns about it.

5. _____ The 24-hour chart check offers nurses the opportunity to find and correct possible medication errors.

Answers: 1. False   2. True   3. True   4. False   5. True

STRATEGIES USED BY NURSES TO PREVENT MEDICATION ERRORS

Nurses have devised various protections against making medication errors. For example, for almost a century they have used the "three-times check" to prevent them from making medication errors. They read the medication cardex, select the medication from the drawer in the medication cart, read the medication label as they place it in a medicine cup, and read it again at the patient's bedside as they prepare to give it to the patient. Furthermore, they concentrate on the "five rights" as a check: the right medication in the right dose is given to the right patient at the right time by the right route of administration. Additional protection is provided as nurses follow the policies and procedures governing medication administration. Nurses do not always read these, since they are not stimulating reading. But the advice included within these books may guard nurses from making errors.

Many nurses use their own rituals as protection. For example, if they have made an error associated with a drug added to an IV, they tend to be very careful and run through a routine before giving that drug again by that route. Another routine involves starting to give medications from the lowest-numbered room that they are responsible for and gradually working up to the highest-numbered room. Nurses are wise to pay attention to their intuitions that tell them that something may not be right about a certain medication order. In that case, it is advisable to stop and check the order.

Another strategy that nurses use to prevent medication errors is reading labels on drug packages carefully. Nurses find themselves picking up lidocaine instead of potassium because the labels are similar. Similar drug names also cause medication errors. And many times nurses do not realize that medications come in different strengths; for example, colace comes in two strengths. In addition, it is advisable to question a sudden and excessive increase in medication dosage and a sudden change to more frequent times of medication administration. These changes signal a potential problem and are worth checking. Also, if nurses find themselves drawing up medication from many vials of injectable medication or pouring out many tablets, this is also a signal that there could be a mistake.

Another warning that a medication error has been made is the accumulation of medications in patient's drawer in the medication cart and the accumulation of bags of refrigerated IVs with medications added in the medication refrigerator. Patients can also be allergic to medications and have cross sensitization to related medications. One example is a penicillin allergy that cross-sensitizes with Keflex (cephalexin monohydrate). Nurses who ask patients if they have ever received a medication before, on finding out that they had not, should be alert for this kind of allergic reactions.

Drug interactions are also difficult to be alert to. Many times nurses are aware of the interactions between drugs that they commonly administer on a specific nursing unit. However, it is difficult to remain knowledgeable about potential drug interactions when new medications are ordered. Also, nurses should check with a hospital pharmacist before crushing medications and mixing them with food for patients who have difficulty swallowing or mixing them with water and giving them through a nasogastric or other tube. Frequently a pharmacist may be able to provide the same medication in a suspension; this modification should also be cleared with the physician, since it alters the original intent of the medication order. Nurses should not automatically assume that if a medication is ordered in tablet form for oral administration that it can be crushed and given via a tube.

Potassium is one medication that deserves special notice, especially when ordered by the IV route. Many medication errors involve potassium chloride (KCl). If KCl is given directly IV, undiluted, cardiac arrest and death can result. Heparin and KCl labels have been very similar in the past, and this labeling has been associated with serious medication errors. Medications that are ordered frequently, such as every 2 hours, are also implicated in medication errors.

It has been suggested that a nurse's chance of making a medication error rate increases on the first or second day back after having some

Exercise 8

List five ways to prevent a medication error.

1. _____

2 _____

3. _____

4. _____

5. _____

Suggested Answers: Three-times check; remaining cognizant of the five rights; getting the physician to order a liquid or suspension instead of crushing a medication; listening to a patient who thinks something is wrong with a medication; being aware of patient allergies; being aware of cross-sensitization; noticing pile-ups of medication; carefully checking original orders against the transcriptions; following hospital policy when taking verbal orders; returning tampered medications or medications with marred labels to pharmacy.

time off. In addition, nurses need to be cautious about medications that are ordered during change-of-shift report. Keeping the response time (time interval between the physician's medication order and the time that the patient receives it) short may help to avoid a medication error. Any medication that is packaged in a defective package or has a blurred or marred label should be returned to the pharmacy. And it is always wise to question orders that are unclear or illegible or that have part of the notation missing.

MEDICATION CALCULATION

Nurses are expected to be able to calculate dosages of medications. Even if a pharmacy follows a unit dose system, situations arise in which the medication available must be measured in order to administer the desired dose.

In order to calculate how much of a medication must be given, nurses can follow this simple formula:

$$\frac{\text{Dose desired}}{\text{Dose on hand}}$$

For example, the physician orders 0.125 mg of Halcion (triazolam). The tablet only comes in 0.250 mg strength.

$$\frac{0.125 \text{ mg}}{0.250 \text{ mg}} = \frac{1}{2} \text{ tablet}$$

Intravenous medications pose another problem. Again, a simple formula is required:

$$\frac{\text{cc/hr}}{60 \text{ mins}} \times \text{drip factor (drops/cc)}$$

For example, a liter of lactated Ringer's solution is ordered to run over 8 hours. The package that contains the IV tubing states: "Drip factor, 10 drops/cc." First, find out the cc per hour by dividing 1000 cc by 8 hours:

$$\frac{1000 \text{ cc}}{8 \text{ hr}} = 125 \text{ cc/hr.}$$

Then, use the above formula:

$$\frac{125 \text{ cc}}{60 \text{ min}} \times \frac{10 \text{ drops}}{\text{cc}} = 20.8, \text{ or } 21 \text{ drops/min.}$$

Mistakes made when performing dosage calculations often lead to medication errors. Common mistakes include: incorrect set-up of the problem; general math mistakes, especially where decimals or fractions are involved; and conversion errors. One conversion error that frequently occurs involves micrograms (mcg) and milligrams (mg). Folic acid, for example, is usually prescribed as 100 mcg (1 mg). Often, it is incorrectly transcribed as 100 mg. The nurse would have to give the patient 100 tablets in order to give 100 milligrams!

Calculation Problems

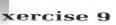xercise 9

1. Hydrocortisone sodium succinate comes in 100 mg/ml vial. You need to give 85 mg IV. How many milliliters of medication would you draw up?

2. Furosemide is prescribed for a small child: 2 mg/kg PO once a day. The child weighs 45 pounds. How much should the child receive? (Hint: 2.2 pounds equals 1 kg.)

3. You need to give your patient 60 mg of gentamicin IV. Gentamicin comes in vials of 40 mg/ml. After adding the drug to a 50-cc bag of dextrose and water, you need to run it at a rate of 50 cc/hour. The drip factor of the IV tubing is 10 drops/cc.
   a. How many milliliters must you draw up?
   b. How many drops per minute will give the appropriate rate?

Answers: 1. 0.85 ml   2. 41 mg   3a. 1.5 ml   3b. 8 drops/min

CONCLUSION

Some medication errors result in harm to patients and are considered very serious mistakes. However, nurses take most errors seriously even if they do not result in harm. They regard them as warnings and institute additional checks and proceed more cautiously. When a medication error takes place, nurses are aware on many levels that the ethical principle to do no harm has been violated. The Nightingale pledge, written in 1893, contains an explicit warning to avoid medication errors. Even though many nurses do not read this code today, they are aware of the message, since it has been repeated over the last ten decades. However, it may be impossible for nurses to avoid making medication errors, even though this is the standard that has been set.

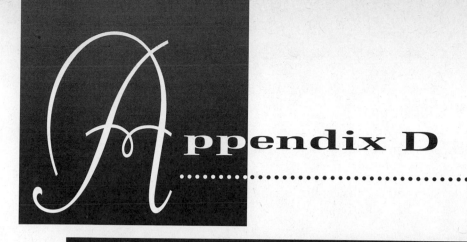

Appendix D

Medication Error Risk-Reduction Test

This test was developed for the study included in Appendix A. The model included in Chapter 11 shaped much of this test. In developing and pretesting this test, I hoped that a sensitive measure of nurses' knowledge of medication errors and risks would be created and revised over time so that nurses who work in hospitals could periodically test their knowledge in this area.

*Consider whether the following items are **true** or **false**. Please circle your answer after reading each test item.*

True/False Test I

1. Medication errors involve patients.	True	False
2. If a physician prescribes a medication incorrectly and a nurse does not question the order, then the nurse is not liable if she or he gives the medication.	True	False
3. Medication errors may involve many hospital departments.	True	False
4. Nurses sometimes give their fellow nurses poor advice about how to deal with the aftermath of a medication error.	True	False
5. One could expect that the more medications a nurse administers, the more likely the chance the nurse will make a medication error.	True	False

6. Lack of standardization in IV medication labeling among manufacturers contributes little to medication errors.   True   False

7. Medication errors are among the most frequent causes of malpractice suits among nurses.   True   False

8. It is considered safe practice to administer oral medication that another nurse or a pharmacist has prepared.   True   False

9. Medication errors involve mistakes of omission and commission.   True   False

10. The "Five Rights" routine and the "three time check" make nurses immune from making medication errors.   True   False

11. One could expect that failure to document a medication error prevents the error from being detected and the nurse from being sued.   True   False

12. It is difficult to get an accurate picture of a hospital's medication error rate because hospital personnel do not often report errors.   True   False

Consider whether the following items are **true** *or* **false**. *Please circle your answer after reading each test item.*

True/False Test II

1. Nurses should question the use of many tablets or vials for a single dose of a medication.   True   False

2. "Zero-error tolerance" rule for medication errors is an achievable goal for a nursing service department.   True   False

3. Nurses should seek other nurses and medical clerk's advice when trying to decipher illegible orders or prescriptions.   True   False

4. Hospital personnel often report medication errors.   True   False

5. When a nurse transcribes a partially legible and incomplete medication order and the patient is seriously harmed, both the nurse and the physician could be liable for malpractice suits.   True   False

6. Procedure manuals report that it is safe to give a medication 1 hour before the time ordered and 1 hour after the time the medication is ordered.   True   False

7. Few patients have the right to refuse to take a medication.   True   False

8. Nurses who witness other nurses pocketing narcotics must report this immediately to a charge nurse or nurse manager.   True   False

9. If a nurse judged it necessary to withhold a medication, then it is sufficient to report it verbally.   True   False

Multiple Choice Test

Circle <u>one</u> best answer to the following questions:

1. The best method of checking a patient's identity in order to ensure that the right patient receives the drug is to:
   1. check the patient's identification band before giving the drug.
   2. go to the patient's bedside and ask the patient his or her name.
   3. check the medication cardex against the medication in the drawer.
   4. double-check the calculation before giving the drug to the patient.

2. It is important to ask another nurse to check the dosages of the following medications in order to prevent medication errors:
   1. anticoagulants and insulins
   2. anticholinergics and antiemetics
   3. antibiotics and antihypertensives
   4. narcotic analgesics and diuretics

3. A handwritten medication order written by a physician should be:
   1. followed if familiar to the nurse who recognizes the medication.
   2. completely recognizable to the nurse transcribing the order.
   3. guessed at by the nurse during an emergency situation.
   4. followed automatically in every situation as written.

4. When taking verbal or oral medication orders from a physician, nurses should:
   1. expect that physicians to state the order slowly and clearly.
   2. question the therapeutic rationale for the medication order.
   3. obtain follow-up information from the physician afterward.
   4. repeat the prescription back to the prescribing physician.

5. When patients question whether they should receive a particular drug, the nurse should:

    1. talk to a pharmacist to determine the appropriateness of the order.

    2. answer any questions the patient has and administer the medication.

    3. review anticipated patient outcomes indicated by the prescription.

    4. double-check the order and drug dispensed before administering it.

Matching Test

Match the categories from the left column (column A) with its corresponding example in the right column (column B). Items in column A may be used more than once in column B.

Column A	Column B
1. Error of omission	RN administers Pavulon, a muscle relaxant, to acutely ill patients so that she or he can play hero.
2. Error of commission	Chemically impaired nurse diverts Demerol for personal use and gives digoxin to patient instead.
3. Criminal act	Pharmacist accidentally mixes aminophylline in excess concentration, IV is administered by a nurse, and an infant dies.

Calculation Problems

Solve the following calculation problems. Include the set-up and the math needed to solve each calculation problem in the space provided.

1. A patient is to receive cimetidine liquid 1200 mg/day in 4 doses. The medication comes in 300 mg/5 ml. How many milliliters would you administer per dose?

2. The physician orders digoxin 0.125 mg IV push at a rate of 0.5 mg/min. Each ampule contains digoxin 0.25 mg/ml. How many milliliters of digoxin would you administer to the patient each minute?

3. A patient is to receive ampicillin 1 gm IM preoperatively. When reconstituting with 0.9 ml of sterile water, a 250-mg vial of ampicillin yields a concentration of 125 mg/0.5 ml. How many milliliters of this reconstituted solution would you administer?

4. A physician orders tobramycin 160 mg IV loading dose to be diluted in 100 ml of normal saline now. Tobramycin vials are labeled: 40 mg/ml. How many milliliters of tobramycin will the nurse add to each 100 ml of normal saline?

5. A patient is to receive 180 mg PO of Procardia daily. Tablets (sustained-release) come in 60 mg tablets. How many tablets will you give at each administration if a patient is to receive the drug q8h?

6. A patient is to receive phenobarbital elixir 240 mg each day. The patient is to receive the phenobarbital in 4 divided doses. Phenobarbital is supplied in 20 mg/ml concentration. How many milliliters of phenobarbital will you give the patient at each dose?

7. An elderly patient receives .375 mg of digoxin elixir every day via a feeding tube. The elixir is supplied .05 mg/ml. How many milliliters will you give at each dose?

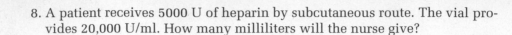

8. A patient receives 5000 U of heparin by subcutaneous route. The vial provides 20,000 U/ml. How many milliliters will the nurse give?

9. A physician orders that a patient is to receive an IV of 1 L of 5% D_5W in 1/2 normal saline solution over 8 hr. What is the drip rate per minute using a 15 drop/ml drip chamber?

$\mathcal{S}$taff Nurse Profile

1. Age:_____

2. Sex: 1. female   2. male

3. Marital status: 1. single
                      2. married
                      3. divorced
                      4. widowed
                      5. separated

4. Highest degree earned: 1. certificate
                           2. diploma
                           3. associate of science in nursing
                           4. other associate's degree
                           5. bachelor of science in nursing
                           6. other bachelor's degree
                           7. master of science in nursing
                           8. master of arts in nursing
                           9. master of business administration
                          10. other master's degree
                          11. doctoral degree
                          12. other, please specify _____

5. Position in nursing: 1. LPN—licensed practical nurse
                           2. RN—staff nurse/charge nurse
                           3. RN—assistant nurse manager
                           4. RN—nurse manager
                           5. RN—other, please specify _____

6. How many medication errors do you remember making over the course of your nursing career? _____

7. How long were you employed at this hospital at the time when you made the medication error that you reported on?_____

8. How long were you employed on the nursing unit where the error occurred? _____

9. What was the total length of your nursing practice experience (the time you actually practiced as a nurse from graduation from your basic program to the time you made the error which you reported) at the time the error occurred?_____

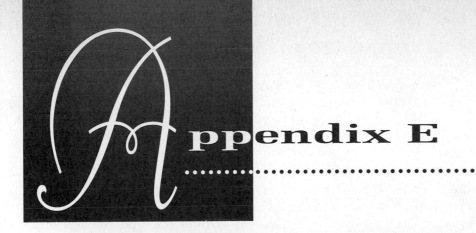

Appendix E

Factors Identified by Nurses as Contributing to Harmful Outcomes from Medication Errors

A Pilot Study

Terry B. McGoldrick
Elaine R. Volk
Frances Warwick
Dalc A. Haakenson
Zane Robinson Wolf

INTRODUCTION

When nurses administer medications, they are committed to upholding an ethical principle: to do good and avoid harm to patients. Although they may not explicitly frame their practice in terms of this principle, they are nevertheless socialized to it in schools of nursing and at work, and they violate it when they make medication errors (Wolf, 1989). Drug errors may be one of the most frequent mistakes nurses make; at times they involve injury and result in lawsuits (Morris, 1981; Poteet, 1983; Springhouse Corp., 1992). The consequences of medication errors include symptoms, scarring, hospitalization (during which the patient is treated to reduce the harm associated with the error), additional treatments and extended length of stay in the hospital if the error is made in the hospital, and death (Jonville, Autret, Bavoux, Bertrand, Barbier & Gauchez, 1991).

Medication errors are mistakes that involve patients and are associated with drugs and intravenous solutions; they are made during the prescription, transcription, dispensing, and administration phases of drug preparation and distribution (Wolf, 1989). These mistakes at work, whether involving a nurse alone or in association with a physician or pharmacist, can jeopardize patient, provider, and institutional safety. "The problems and sources of medication errors are multidisciplinary and multifactorial" (American Society of Hospital Pharmacists, 1992, p. 640).

System-originated medication errors, such as those involving confusing drug labels, can be corrected. But random errors—those that happen by chance and without an evident pattern—are difficult to eliminate (Elnicki & Schmitt, 1980; Hassall & Daniels, 1983). In spite of retrospective and prospective efforts by nurses, risk managers, and other hospital personnel, it may be impossible to eliminate them. Nevertheless, nurses share the responsibility to reduce and eliminate such errors.

The purpose of this study is to describe and explain factors identified by nurses as contributing to the outcome of patient harm following the commission of medication errors resulting from medication errors made by registered nurses (RNs) and licensed practical nurses (LPNs). The factors are (1) phase of preparation and administration, (2) indicators contributing to the error, (3) interventions needed as a result of the error, and (4) type of position and number of staff responsible for making the error. The investigators will survey RNs and LPNs who may have made medication errors using the Medication Error Risk Profile (MERP), a self-report instrument (Wolf, 1989, 1992).

In this research, phase of preparation and administration is defined as the stage of medication administration from prescription to administration during which a medication error may be made; indicator contributing to the possible error is defined as the fact that signals the occurrence of a medication error, such as wrong dose or wrong time. Interventions needed as a result of the error is defined as the nursing or medical action aimed at detecting or reducing the potential or actual harm incurred from the medication error, while type of position and number of staff responsible for making the medication error are the category of hospital employee involved in the error and the total number of those employees involved in the error.

REVIEW OF THE LITERATURE

Nurses are keenly aware that they serve "as the final checkpoint in the system" for dispensing medication (Adams & Burleson, 1992, p. 951) and rely on personal and professional rituals, hospital procedures, and advice to prevent them from making errors (Kaplan, 1991; Springhouse Corp., 1991; Wolf, 1986, 1992). At times preventive strategies fail, leaving many distressed by their mistakes and searching for tactics to prevent future errors.

Since patient harm can result from medication errors, and harm is considered the worst-case scenario for hospital nursing practice, nurse administrators take the position that only no errors are acceptable. However, this zero-tolerance standard may be impossible to realize (Manthey, 1989) and may result simply in reducing the number of errors reported by nurses.

Actions to prevent medication errors are published in hospital policies and procedures; nursing staff are introduced to these standards of care during orientation sessions. Risk management departments in health care institutions are also targeted to eliminate harm to patients, personnel, and the agency and to reduce the cost associated with unusual events or incidents, such as medication errors (Poteet, 1983). Furthermore, nurses have created rules and ritualistic checks to keep them from making medication errors. These serve to help nurses focus on the task at hand when surrounded by distractions (Hodgkin, 1984; Ludwig-Beymer et al., 1990; Springhouse Corp., 1992).

Nursing service organizations have developed point systems to evaluate medication errors, along with protocols to determine disciplinary actions (Cobb, 1990; Lowery, 1991) and severity indexes to determine actions to take following errors (Brandt, Deml, Gerke & Lee, 1988; Walters et al., 1992). These approaches are intended to ensure more uniform handling of medication errors and may positively influence the rate of reporting medication errors. More systematic classification and weighing of medication errors could increase awareness of causative factors among nurses and result in reduced error rates and more consistent follow-up. However, some nurses believe that point systems might inhibit reporting of medication errors rather than serve to prevent errors.

After making a medication error, many nurses feel guilty and may expect or desire some form of punishment or reparation as payment for their mistake (Wolf, 1989, 1992). Others fear punishment, which may vary from the "emotional pain of shame and guilt" (Manthey, 1989a, p. 19) to more public forms of humiliation and termination from their jobs. Manthey (1989) suggested that discipline and punishment are synonymous to nurses. However, the terms are not synonymous since punishment causes pain, whereas discipline maintains order. Subsequently, Manthey (1989b) proposed that nonpunitive responses to mistakes at work provide the wrongdoer with the opportunity to gain knowledge and skill and to revise attitudes about medication errors. Providing corrective action that involves education may result in nurses' reporting more medication errors, since the action taken is no longer seen as punitive. Since human error can only be reduced, not eliminated, McClure (1991) has suggested that nursing needs to become more forgiving of these errors while demanding corrective action, especially when patient safety is threatened. A medication error does not automatically imply incompetence.

Medication errors are made during different phases or stages of preparation and administration. For example, various authors (American Society of Hospital Pharmacists (ASHP), 1992; Betz & Levy, 1985) have characterized types of errors according to the dispensing, prescribing, transcription, and administration phases. Indicators that point to or describe errors are identified often in the literature and include unordered medication, wrong dose of medication, wrong route of administration of medication, and omission of a medication dose (ASHP, 1992; Betz & Levy, 1985; Cobb, 1990; Fuqua & Stevens, 1988; Poster & Pelletier, 1988). Hospitals frequently classify medication errors by such terms.

Following medication errors, hospital staff act to prevent harm or to limit it (Jonville et al., 1991); these interventions are described as corrective or supportive (ASHP, 1992). Diagnostic studies are ordered, medications are given, and vital signs are monitored. Furthermore, it is generally acknowledged that medication errors are multidisciplinary and are committed by pharmacists, physicians, nurses, pharmacy technicians, students, ward clerk, and others (ASHP, 1992; Fuqua & Stevens, 1988; Markowitz, Pearson, Kay & Lowenstein, 1981; McNeilly, 1987).

Jonville et al. (1991) conducted a six-month prospective study with 16 poison control centers in France in order to describe the epidemiology of medication errors in pediatric patients. The consequences of the 1222 reported medication errors were evaluated; they included hospitalization, scarring, and death. When children were hospitalized as a result of the errors, they demonstrated symptoms and were treated with various modalities, including gastric evacuation, assisted ventilation, and medications to manage overdoses. Physicians and nurses committed most of the errors that took place in hospitals, while members of the family and pharmacists made those outside the hospital. The investigators pointed out that reported medication errors fail to give an accurate picture of actual drug-related mistakes, since errors that do not involve clinical symptoms are often not reported.

Davis, Hoyt, McArdle, Mackersie, Shackford & Eastman (1991) investigated the contributions of critical care errors to mortality and morbidity in six designated trauma centers in the United States. Preventable errors were identified in 670 of 12,910 patients who were admitted to the centers. Errors included errors in management, monitoring errors, drug and electrolyte errors, and procedural/technical errors. Examples of types of injuries resulting from drug and electrolyte errors included central nervous system injury, hyperkalemia, and hypersensitivity reaction. Drug and electrolyte errors were the cause of preventable deaths (injuries/sequelae considered survivable or care suspect, directly or indirectly caused death) in three patients.

Kuehm and Doyle (1990), of the Risk Prevention Department of the Medical Inter-Insurance Exchange of New Jersey, analyzed 337 files in which medication error was a significant cause of suits from 1977 to 1988. Indemnities were paid due to medication errors in these cases; medication error was the chief cause of suit in 57 percent of these files. In the remaining 43 percent of the files, medication error was an important factor. Allergic reaction, error in writing the prescription, communication failure, administration of excessive dosage of medication, prescription of contraindicated medication, failure to monitor drugs for toxic levels, treatment with antibiotics, prescription of medication to treat symptoms, and generic drugs are the nine reported categories of actions that indicated trends in malpractice claims. Patients involved in the suits were reported to have suffered morbidity and death as a result of errors. Examples of injuries included profound brain damage, addiction to pain medication, amputation of limbs, some degree of hearing loss, and decreased visual acuity.

In a 4-year prospective quality assurance study (Raju, Kecskes, Thornton, Perry & Feldman, 1989), 315 iatrogenic medication errors were reported among 2147 neonatal and pediatric intensive care admissions; the error rate was 1 per 6.8 admissions. "Patient injuries were classified into four categories: 1 = no apparent injury; 2 = mild injury, when the injury required no substantial treatment or intervention; 3 = potentially serious injury, when the drug serum level was in the toxic range with a potential for serious consequences or physiological side-effects in an otherwise symptom-free patient, or when an insufficient dose of a life-saving drug had been given; and 4 = substantial injury, when a long-term injury occurred with extension of the hospital stay by a day or more or when there were signs and symptoms of toxic effects of a drug, or if the patient died as a result of the medication error" (Raju et al., 1989, p. 374). Errors were more frequent on the day shift, were most often attributed to nurses, and frequently involved the medication's being given at the wrong time. Patient injuries included extravasation of intravenous solutions into tissues and resulting in local tissue damage, hyperglycemia, inadequate sedation, loss of a central venous catheter, and tachycardia, tachypnea, and excessive sweating. The investigators were certain that most errors that resulted in patient injury were reported. However, they acknowledged that when voluntary reporting systems were in place, errors were not always reported. The investigators encouraged hospitals to develop nonpunitive longitudinal monitoring systems. Different classification schemes have been identified to assist nurses and other health care providers to assess harm to the patient (ASHP, 1992). However, no studies were located identifying variables that predict patient harm following medication errors.

Brandt, Deml, Gerke, and Lee (1988) categorized the severity of medication incidents according to the actions that should be taken following medication errors. Category I errors required little or no medical or nursing intervention; category II incidents produced systemic or localized responses requiring intervention to counteract medications or flow rates; and category III incidents were potentially life-threatening and required immediate medical and nursing intervention to counteract reactions (p. 801). While the authors did not investigate the relationships among medication error indicators and severity or patient harm, they did advise nurses to examine trends in medication errors and follow-up care.

CONCEPTUAL ORIENTATION

Hughes (1951) suggested that occupations are constituted by bundles of skills, some of which "require more repetition than others for the original learning and for maintenance" (p. 320). He proposed that one common theme is that of the mistakes and failures that members of an occupation make as they practice their skills at work.

Nurses' mistakes, similar to those of pharmacists and physicians, can be more harmful than those of other occupations because of the human, personal care aspects of their occupation. When a medication error occurs, not only personal but departmental and institutional risks are evident, as are the risk-dispersing devices used by nurses. As the mistake unfolds, nurses put into use the "collective rationale which they whistle to one another to keep up their courage" (Hughes, 1951, p. 321). Often the mistake is "owned" in a corporate sense by the nurses directly and indirectly involved in the medication error (Wolf, 1986).

Wolf (1989) constructed a model to explain risks, types, and patient consequences of nurse-made medication errors. The model was generated from Wolf's (1986) ethnographic study of nursing rituals, since nurse informants in the study classified types and variations in the types of medication errors, and from the literature reviewed for an article on medication errors (Wolf, 1989). It was recently revised as a result of other studies on medication errors, using phenomenological, focus group, and story-telling methods (Wolf, 1992). (See Figure 10-1). The model was used to generate a medication error checklist aimed at eliciting descriptions of medication errors and gauging the risks associated with them.

METHODS

The investigators will use the Medication Error Risk Profile (MERP) to survey nurses in order to describe factors identified by nurses as contributing to a harmful outcome resulting from nurse-made medication errors. Scores on the criterion variable patient harm will be computed using the data reported on the Visual Analog Degree of Harm Scale (VAS), which will be measured from left to right using the nearest millimeter. Phases of preparation and administration, factors intrinsic to and leading to the error, interventions needed as a result of the error, and hospital staff responsible for making the error will also be described. Phases of preparation and administration will be entered into a forced entry regression equations as dummy variables as will the type of position of hospital staff making the error. The number and percent of factors intrinsic to and leading to errors will be described as will the nursing and medical interventions use to care for patients following the errors. The type of position of hospital staff responsible for making the error and the total number of staff responsible for making the error will also be described.

INSTRUMENTATION

Data on criterion and predictor variables will be elicited on the MERP, which was created using the health care agency incident model and the literature on medication errors from nursing, medicine, and pharmacology as guides to generate items and to provide content validity (Lynn, 1986). Variables included in the instrument and constituting the content domain were derived largely from the literature on factors associated with medication errors and through the model. Items were revised and rearranged following suggestions by nurses working at staff nurse, staff development instructor, nurse manager, clinical director, and chief nurse executive levels.

Furthermore, content validity of the MERP was established by a chief nurse executive, two clinical directors of nursing, two nurse managers, one quality assurance coordinator and one risk manager, both of whom are nurses, and two staff nurses. A physician and a pharmacist provided expert validation. Experts rated appropriateness of items on the instrument, as well as the clarity (clear/unclear) of each item on the MERP. They also evaluated the clarity of the directions to guide respondents to complete the instrument.

Following revision, the investigators established the interobserver reliability of the instrument by having two master's-prepared nurses, a quality assurance coordinator and a director of nursing, who independently ranked two medication error incidents using the MERP. Pearson correlation coefficients were calculated on the judges' ratings of both medication errors using the instrument; both resulted in strong correlations ($r = .81$, $p = .000$; $r = .78$, $p = > .05$).

Part I of the MERP contains questions regarding the location and time of the medication error, the day of the week the error occurred, the medication involved in the error, the VAS estimating the degree of harm resulting from the error, and the health care workers and departments notified of the error. Part II includes items encouraging subjects to classify the error as error of commission or omission. Part III is an indicator checklist containing the phases of preparation and administration when the error took place and the indicators contributing to the error. Included in part IV was a question encouraging subjects to describe actions taken after the error was discovered. Also in this section were items on interventions needed as a result of the error and hospital staff positions (RN, LPN, pharmacist, physician, etc.) representing individuals responsible for the error and the hours worked by such individuals. The following scale was used in parts II, III, and IV of the MERP: yes = 1; no = 0. A staff nurse profile will also be used and includes questions regarding nurse demographics.

SAMPLE AND PROCEDURES FOR DATA COLLECTION

RNs and LPNs who are currently employed in health care agencies will be asked to participate in a survey in which the MERP is used as a self-report instrument to help them describe a medication error that they may have made within the past year. Names of RNs and LPNs who may be contacted will be obtained through employee lists from three hospitals and from an enrollment list from a university school of nursing with an RN-BSN program. Two hundred subjects will be sought by a systematic random sampling technique.

It is assumed that subjects who have made medication errors will complete the survey. Subjects will be invited to participate in the study via a letter and asked to complete the MERP. They will be encouraged to mail completed instruments to the investigators in self-addressed, stamped envelopes. Consent to participate in the study will be indicated as each respondent completes the instrument. Confidentiality and anonymity of subjects will be assured. No names of nurses, patients, physicians, pharmacists, employees, hospitals, health care agencies, or other institutions will be recorded on the MERP. The nursing research committee and institutional review board of one hospital and an institutional review board of a university will be asked to review and approve of the study.

DATA ANALYSIS

Descriptive statistics on subject characteristics and factors included on the MERP will be calculated using SPSS-x, version 3.

$\int$ ample Letter

The following letter will be used to recruit nurses to participate in this research study. It has been carefully worded to provide complete anonymity to the participants.

Dear Nurse:

We would like to invite you to participate anonymously in a research study.

Names were randomly selected from a list of actively employed nurses or from a list of RN-BSN and MSN students provided by a university. This letter is the only contact we will have with you. Your anonymous input will be kept confidential.

The purpose of this study is to determine the contributions of certain factors to patient harm following a potential medication error. You will be asked to complete a survey using the Medication Error Risk Profile (MERP). We will use your responses to determine factors that may contribute to patient harm following possible medication errors.

When you read the MERP, I would like you to think about a possible medication error that you may have made in the past year and can remember vividly. Please complete the survey with this event in mind. Do not sign the enclosed forms. Additionally, do not identify yourself, your hospital, your university, your colleagues, the patient, or anyone associated with the event in any manner whatsoever.

Please insert the completed instrument in the enclosed stamped envelope.

Thank you for your help.

Sincerely,

Zane Robinson Wolf, PhD, RN, FAAN

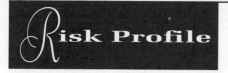

Medication Error Risk Profile

Part I: Demographic Profile of Medication Error Event

1. Department where medication error occurred: _____

2. Unit where medication error occurred: _____

3. Time medication error discovered:_____ AM _____ PM

4. Time medication error occurred: _____

5. Circle day of week medication error occurred:

   Monday   Wednesday   Friday   Sunday

   Tuesday   Thursday   Saturday

6. Identify the medication(s) involved in the error:

   _____

   _____

   _____

   _____

7. Rate the degree of harm resulting from this medication error. Let the rating represent your own clinical judgment. Make a vertical mark through the horizontal line.

   (No Harm) _____ (Extremely Harmful)

8. Circle "yes" or "no" as to health care workers and department(s) who were notified of the medication error:

8.1	Attending physician:	Yes	No
8.2	Resident physician:	Yes	No
8.3	Director of nursing:	Yes	No
8.4	Nurse manager:	Yes	No
8.5	Risk manager:	Yes	No
8.6	Pharmacist:	Yes	No
8.7	Patient:	Yes	No
8.8	Other:	Yes	No

Part II: Medication Error Classification

1. This medication error was an error of omission   Yes   No
   (an error of omission is a medication error in which
   the prescribed medication is not given).

2. This medication error was an error of commission   Yes   No
   (an error of commission is a medication error in which
   a medication that was not prescribed is given).

Part III: Medication Error Indicator Checklist

1. Circle "yes" or "no" as to the phase(s) of preparation and administration during
   which the medication error took place:

1.1 Prescription	Yes	No
1.2 Dispensing	Yes	No
1.3 Distribution	Yes	No
1.4 Transcription	Yes	No
1.5 Administration	Yes	No

Directions: Please answer each item by circling your response using both scales that are
provided.

This medication error involved the following indicators which contributed to the error:

     Yes = 1
     No = 0

Rank this medication error indicator in relation to how much it contributed to seriousness of the error.

     0 = does not apply
     1 = did not contribute
     2 = contributed minimally
     3 = contributed moderately
     4 = contributed greatly

1. Wrong drug	Yes	No	0	1	2	3	4
2. Wrong dose	Yes	No	0	1	2	3	4
3. Dose calculation incorrect	Yes	No	0	1	2	3	4
4. Wrong route	Yes	No	0	1	2	3	4
5. Wrong time	Yes	No	0	1	2	3	4
6. Extra dose	Yes	No	0	1	2	3	4
7. Medication not ordered	Yes	No	0	1	2	3	4
8. Out of sequence	Yes	No	0	1	2	3	4
9. Discontinued	Yes	No	0	1	2	3	4
10. Unclear order	Yes	No	0	1	2	3	4

11. Improper order	Yes	No	0	1	2	3	4
12. Order not written on physician order sheet	Yes	No	0	1	2	3	4
13. Order not written on medication cardex	Yes	No	0	1	2	3	4
14. Medication transcribed incorrectly	Yes	No	0	1	2	3	4
15. Order recopied incorrectly on cardex	Yes	No	0	1	2	3	4
16. Medication overlooked	Yes	No	0	1	2	3	4
17. Medication misread	Yes	No	0	1	2	3	4
18. Previous dose not documented	Yes	No	0	1	2	3	4
19. Incorrect documentation	Yes	No	0	1	2	3	4
20. Unrenewed medication given	Yes	No	0	1	2	3	4
21. Expired medication given	Yes	No	0	1	2	3	4
22. Known allergy, medication given	Yes	No	0	1	2	3	4
23. Adverse reaction unrecognized at first	Yes	No	0	1	2	3	4
24. Medication mislabeled	Yes	No	0	1	2	3	4
25. Medication missing	Yes	No	0	1	2	3	4
26. Wrong medication sent	Yes	No	0	1	2	3	4
27. Medication given before blood test or culture taken	Yes	No	0	1	2	3	4
28. Medication given before drug blood level drawn	Yes	No	0	1	2	3	4
29. Medication given that others prepare	Yes	No	0	1	2	3	4
30. Wrong dosage form	Yes	No	0	1	2	3	4
31. Outdated medication given	Yes	No	0	1	2	3	4
32. Incorrect route of administration used such as IM, PO, or IV	Yes	No	0	1	2	3	4

33. Wrong IV solution	Yes	No	0	1	2	3	4
34. Wrong IV rate of flow	Yes	No	0	1	2	3	4
35. Pump malfunction	Yes	No	0	1	2	3	4
36. Incorrect pump setting	Yes	No	0	1	2	3	4
37. Site problem	Yes	No	0	1	2	3	4

38. This error was a systems (methods by which medications are prescribed, dispensed, administered in hospital) error   Yes   No

39. This error was a random (by chance) error   Yes   No

Part IV: Follow-up

Objective description of action taken after medication error discovered:

_____

_____

_____

_____

Circle "yes" or "no" as to interventions needed as a result of the error:

1. Additional medication administered as a result of error.   Yes   No

    Please specify medication administered _____

2. Additional laboratory studies done as result of error.   Yes   No

    Please specify additional laboratory studies _____

3. Radiology studies done as a result of error.   Yes   No

    Please specify radiology studies _____

4. Symptoms related to error.   Yes   No

    Please specify symptoms _____

5. Patient transferred to another unit.   Yes   No

    Please specify unit _____

6. Extra nursing time spent monitoring patient as result of error. Yes No

   Please specify extra nursing time _____

7. Extra length of stay as a result of error. Yes No

   Please specify additional length of stay _____

Responsibility for Medication Error

1. Registered nurse	Yes	No
2. Licensed practical nurse	Yes	No
3. Nursing assistant	Yes	No
4. Medical clerk	Yes	No
5. Professional nursing student	Yes	No
6. Practical nursing student	Yes	No
7. Pharmacist	Yes	No
8. Physician	Yes	No
9. Patient	Yes	No
10. Patient's family	Yes	No
11. Other	Yes	No

12. In the two-day period prior to the error, how many total hours were worked at any hospital or location by the responsible person or persons?

Position of person involved   Number of hours worked

_____   _____

_____   _____

_____   _____

Rank the degree of harm that resulted from the medication error. Please use the scale provided and circle your response:

0 = no harmful effect (improvement in symptoms, condition; no change in symptoms or condition).

1 = moderately harmful effect (morbidity: symptoms, illness)

2 = severely harmful effect (morbidity: severe symptoms, permanent disability)

3 = maximally harmful effect (mortality: death)

⨍taff Nurse Profile

1. Age: _____

2. Sex: 1. female   2. male

3. Marital status:
   1. single
   2. married
   3. divorced
   4. widowed
   5. separated

4. Highest degree earned:
   1. certificate
   2. diploma
   3. associate of science in nursing
   4. other associate's degree
   5. bachelor of science in nursing
   6. other bachelor's degree
   7. master of science in nursing
   8. master of arts in nursing
   9. master of business administration
   10. other master's degree
   11. doctoral degree
   12. other, please specify _____

5. Position in nursing:
   1. LPN—licensed practical nurse
   2. RN—staff nurse/charge nurse
   3. RN—assistant nurse manager
   4. RN—nurse manager
   5. RN—other, please specify _____

6. How many medication errors do you remember making over the course of your nursing career? _____

7. How long (in months) were you employed at this hospital at the time when you made the medication error that you reported?_____

8. How long (in months) were you employed on the nursing unit where the error occurred?_____

9. What was the total length of your nursing practice experience (in months) (the time you actually practiced as a nurse from graduation from your basic program to the time you made the error which you reported) at the time the error occurred? _____

REFERENCES

Adams, T. D., & Burleson, K. W. (1992). Continuous quality improvement in a medication error reporting system. *P & T*, (June), 943–951.

American Society of Hospital Pharmacists Council on Professional Affairs. (1992). Draft guidelines on preventable medication errors. *AJHP, 49*, 640–648.

Betz, R. P., & Levy, H. B. (1985). An interdisciplinary method of classifying and monitoring medication errors. *American Journal of Hospital Pharmacy, 42,* 1724–1732.

Brandt, M., Deml, M., Gerke, M. L., & Lee, E. H. (1988). A severity index for medication errors. *Nursing Management, 19*(8), 80I–80P.

CSHP Committee. (1986). CSHP guidelines for medication incident and medication discrepancy reporting in Canadian hospital. *Canadian Journal of Hospital Pharmacy, 39*(3), 67–69.

Cobb, M. D. (1990). Dealing fairly with medication errors. *Nursing '90* (March), 42–42.

Davis, J. W., Hoyt, D. B., McArdle, M. S., Mackersie, R. C., Shackford, S. R., & Eastman, A. B. (1991). The significance of critical care errors in causing preventable death in trauma patients in a trauma system. *Journal of Trauma, 31*(6), 813–819.

Elnicki, R. A., & Schmitt, J. P. (1980). Contributions of patient and hospital characteristics to adverse incidents. *Health Services Research, 15*, 398–414.

Fuqua, R. A., & Stevens, K. R. (1988). What we know about medication errors: A literature review. *Journal of Nursing Quality Assurance, 3*(1), 1–17.

Groff, J. (1896). Hand-book of materia medica for trained nurses. *Trained Nurse, 16*, 635–640.

Haley, S. M., & Osberg, J. S. (1989). Kappa coefficient calculation using multiple ratings per subject: A special communication. *Physical Therapy, 69*(11), 970–974.

Hassall, T. H., & Daniels, C. E. (1983). Evaluation of three types of control chart methods in unit dose error monitoring. *American Journal of Hospital Pharmacy, 40*(6), 970–975.

Hodgin, L. (1984). Sarnia General develops medication error report. *Dimensions in Health Service, 61*(3), 25–43.

Hughes, E. C. (1951). Mistakes at work. *Journal of Economics and Political Science, 17*, 320–327.

Jonville, A. E., Autret, E., Bavoux, F., Bertrand, P. P., Barbier, P., & Gauchez, A. M. (1991). Characteristics of medication errors in pediatric. *DICP, The Annals of Pharmacotherapy, 25*, 1113–1117.

Kaplan, M. J. (1991). *Experiences of registered nurses and physicians with making medication errors.* Master's thesis, La Salle University, Philadelphia, PA.

Kuehm, S. L., & Doyle, M. J. (1990). Medication errors: 1977 to 1988. *New Jersey Medicine, 87*(1), 27–34.

Lowery, K. (1991). *Medication error prevention through trending and reporting of errors.* Grand View Hospital, Quality Assurance Department, Grand View, PA.

Ludwig-Beymer, P., Czurylo, K. T., Gattuso, M. C., Hennessy, K. A., & Ryan, C. J. (1990). The effect of testing on the reported incidence of medication errors in a medical center. *Journal of Continuing Education in Nursing, 21*(1), 11–17.

Lynn, M. L. (1986). Determination and quantification of content validity. *Nursing Research, 35*(6), 382–385.

Manthey, M. (1989a). Discipline without punishment—Part I. *Nursing Management* (October), 19.

Manthey, M. (1989b). Discipline without punishment—Part II. *Nursing Management* (November), 23.

Markowitz, J. S., Pearson, G., Kay, B. G., & Lowenstein, R. (1981). Nurses, physicians, and pharmacists: Their knowledge of hazards of medications. *Nursing Research, 30*(6), 366–370.

McClure, M. L. (1991). Human error—A professional dilemma. *Journal of Professional Nursing, 7*(4), 207.

McNeilly, J. L. (1987). Medication errors: A quality assurance tool. *Nursing Management, 18*(12), 53–58.

Morris, W. O. (1981). The negligent nurse—the physician and the hospital. *Baylor Law Review, 33*(1), 109–143.